I0819013

The Menopause Gut

THE Menopause Gut

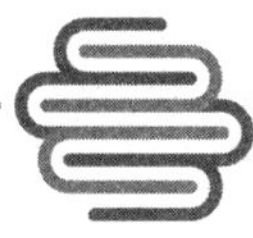

Balance Your Microbiome to Reclaim Your Health in Midlife and Beyond

CYNTHIA THURLOW, NP

AVERY
an imprint of Penguin Random House
New York

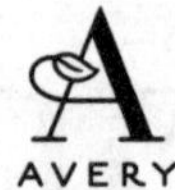

AVERY
an imprint of Penguin Random House LLC
1745 Broadway, New York, NY 10019
penguinrandomhouse.com

Most Avery books are available at a discount when purchased in quantity for sales promotions or corporate use. Special editions, which include personalized covers, excerpts, and corporate imprints, can be created when purchased in large quantities. For more information, please email specialmarkets@penguinrandomhouse.com. Your local bookstore can also assist with discounted bulk purchases using the Penguin Random House corporate Business-to-Business program. For assistance in locating a participating retailer, email B2B@penguinrandomhouse.com.

Book design by Lorie Pagnozzi

Library of Congress Cataloging-in-Publication Data has been applied for.

ISBN 9780593855195
eBook ISBN 9780593855201

Printed in the United States of America
1st Printing

The authorized representative in the EU for product safety and compliance is Penguin Random House Ireland, Morrison Chambers, 32 Nassau Street, Dublin D02 YH68, Ireland, https://eu-contact.penguin.ie.

To my three favorite humans: my husband, Todd; my boys, Jack and Liam; and, of course, the doods, Cooper, Baxter, and Hamilton. Everything I do in my life is in honor of you.

And to all my female patients over the past twenty-five years, thank you for inspiring me to do the true work I was put on this earth to do: educate, inspire, and empower women in middle age and beyond.

Contents

Introduction

My Own Midlife Pause

It started out as an incredibly romantic getaway. In September 2018, my husband, Todd, and I splurged on a trip to Morocco and southern Spain for our fifteenth wedding anniversary. First stop: Marrakech, which was everything I imagined it would be—exotic, hot, and exploding with color and light. As with other trips out of the country, we were both very conscientious about where we ate and drank, as it's not uncommon to get food poisoning while traveling. After Marrakech, it was on to Casablanca, where we spent the night before traveling to Nerja in southern Spain. This is where the story starts to go downhill: In the middle of the first night in Spain, I woke up to the worst vomiting I'd ever experienced in my entire life. It was so bad that at one point, I worried that all the forceful vomiting would tear my esophagus (called a Mallory-Weiss tear; sometimes, knowing so much about the body can be a blessing and a curse). Unfortunately, I was also having diarrhea—I was battling this on both ends. Every time I went back to bed, I would need the bathroom again, so I finally acquiesced and lay down on the tiled floor next to the shower. In between bouts, I wondered why I was so sick but my husband wasn't—we'd both eaten the same thing the previous evening. *What was making me so ill?* We were supposed to go to the Alhambra the next day—a famous Moorish palace I had always dreamed of visiting, especially its Patio of the Lions. And all I could think of, in between retches, was how I needed to feel better so I could make it there.

By sunup the next morning, the violent retching had stopped, and so, too, the diarrhea. I certainly didn't feel 100 percent, but I was determined to make it to the palace. I got in the car with Todd, who drove (thank you, babe, as I was in no shape to drive in a foreign country) the winding roads from our hotel in Nerja to the Alhambra, about an hour away. (Let me tell you, it did not disappoint.) As the days passed, we continued to sightsee around southern Spain, and I could gradually eat something more substantive besides bone broth, water, and electrolytes. For the rest of the trip, I kept myself hydrated and tried to rest as much as possible. I chalked up the experience to yet another bad bout of food poisoning and didn't really give it much thought. I mean, *what else could it have been?*

Cut to a few months later, in December 2018, when I traveled to Toronto to give my first TEDx talk. I was ecstatic to be there but also nervous. The night before the speech, I went around the corner from the hotel to an organic store and picked up a big salad with chicken (good protein in prep for my big day). I ate, drank a lot of water, and went to bed. I woke up with my stomach doing somersaults, and I had loose stools, but I was convinced it was related to nerves; it's not uncommon to have a little bit of GI upset when nervous or anxious about something. I was well prepped—I had the talk committed to memory—but those anxious feelings always popped up when I spoke in front of strangers. I nailed my talk—and chided myself for being so nervous beforehand. I went home and forgot all about my stomach upset, until I was talking to my functional medicine provider. He told me, "Well, you realize there was this huge *E. coli* outbreak in Toronto while you were there." Eek.

I got tested, and it was confirmed: I had acute *E. coli*. We addressed it with antimicrobials (supplements with a potent ability to kill off the bacteria), and that was that—or so I thought. Two months later, I accompanied my husband on a business trip to Hawaii. (I swear my life is not always this glamorous!) I was home for about twenty-four hours when I woke up in the middle of the night to another horrible episode of diarrhea and vomiting. *What the heck is going on? I thought I got rid of the* E. coli. *Do I just have the worst luck?* I thought. I initially blamed food poisoning again, but I spent the next day in bed, and by late afternoon, when I wasn't feeling any better, I texted a fellow nurse practitioner and friend, who suggested I go to the hospital.

"If you're having abdominal pain and can't keep fluids down, you need to get this checked out, Cynthia. You know that, right?" she said.

She was right—I needed to go. So I went to the ER, but by that point, I was in so much pain, I could not get comfortable. (Believe me, it was worse than labor.) I couldn't lie still on the stretcher; I kept squirming when they tried to take my vital signs. The nurse and physician assistant could clearly see I was in excruciating pain, but they didn't make much of my story or symptoms initially, as my vital signs showed no signs of distress. Scratching their heads, they gave me Maalox in desperation, but it didn't help. A morbid thought entered my mind: *What if they don't figure out what's wrong with me? Am I going to die?* I had an impending sense of doom—that something significant was happening in my body, although it wasn't clear to me what that was. And then my blood work came back, and that's when things started to happen very quickly. I got upgraded to the lead ER physician, who ordered a CT scan of my abdomen and pelvis stat. When she reviewed the scan, she told me, "You have a ruptured appendix and pancolitis [inflammation of the colon]." She brought in a surgeon, who wanted to operate that evening and take out a portion of my colon.

"Whoa," I said. "No one's taking my colon." While I was surprised that I had appendicitis—most cases are in younger people—I was more concerned about losing part of a vital organ unnecessarily. That would mean getting a colostomy, even if it was only temporary.

As sick as I was, I knew that taking my colon would be a very, very bad idea. The doctors coalesced and started me on multiple antibiotics and antifungals, and I was placed on an NG—a nasogastric tube that is fed through your nose into your stomach—to decompress my evolving list of complications, which included a small-bowel obstruction. After thirteen days of hospitalization riddled with complications—I had lost fifteen pounds, and my body was starting to catabolize my muscles—I was discharged from the hospital. The plan was to have my appendix removed in six weeks after I healed a bit, so I went home with a central line (a special IV to administer outpatient medications). I looked like a skeleton and felt like one, too. I had no energy.

My medical team, which consisted of three specialists, the surgeon, an infectious disease specialist, and a gastroenterologist, put me on six weeks of IV antibiotics and antifungals. Every week, I would go to the interventional radiologist's imaging center to see if I was ready to have a drain removed that was situated between my cecum (part of my large intestine) and my inflamed appendix. You see, among my myriad complications, I had developed a fistula, which is a tunnel that connects two parts of our bodies that should not otherwise be connected. In the meantime, I had previously committed to doing a second TEDx talk. The folks who ran it had no idea I had been in the hospital. I was doing better—I could eat and sleep. My surgeon signed off on my trip to and from Greenville, South Carolina, provided I was not having more symptoms. (I am so glad I did, even with a ruptured appendix—that second TEDx talk, about intermittent fasting, now has more than fifteen million views and has changed my career trajectory.) Ten days later, I had my appendix out.

My gastric emergency was finally "over." I was no longer in the hospital fighting for my life or dealing with the horrific complications—but what I didn't know at that time was that I had not truly gotten to the root cause of my illnesses. That took a conversation in early 2020 with Dr. Gabrielle Lyon (who would go on to publish the bestseller *Forever Strong*). I met her for the first time on a panel, and we became fast friends. In one conversation, I had told her about my recent health fiasco.

"Hmmm . . . I know you were on some great trips—tell me where you traveled in the last year or so," she said.

"Well, I got *E. coli* in Toronto, and before that, I'd been in Morocco, where I picked up some other stomach bug."

"You know, I take care of a lot of special-ops guys in my practice, and you and your husband have traveled places many people haven't. I think you picked up giardia when you were in Morocco," she told me. "And that kept your immune system both over-activated and compromised, which can lead to a secondary infection and appendicitis."

She was right. I got tested for giardia—a parasite known to be prevalent in that area of North Africa—and it was still in my system. I was put on antibiotics for that and it cleared it up. The bug went away, but the lasting impacts didn't. As a nurse practitioner and hormone expert who has advised thousands of women on their health journeys, I felt compelled to figure out *how* I got giardia and *E. coli* in the first place so that I could better keep myself and my patients healthy. Over time and after much research, I have an unexpected answer for you: perimenopause. While it was giardia that put me in the hospital with a slew of complications, my being in perimenopause started it all. Why is that?

And if I didn't know then, how could I expect my patients and clients to know?

Like most women, I didn't think too much about it when I was forty-seven, in 2018. I wasn't aware that I was fully in perimenopause because it had creeped up on me. And like most women, when they see a healthcare provider about their symptoms, they often don't know much more than "This is just part of being a woman" or "We all get older." Symptoms may be the usual suspects: hot flashes, mood swings, night sweats, low libido, memory issues, and weight gain. The not-so-usual suspects: joint pain, dry eye, itchy skin or ear canals, and frozen shoulder. Worse, we were told we could do nothing about them: "That's life." With so little research that has been done historically on women in perimenopause and menopause, it isn't surprising. But traditional medicine that has belittled female menopausal symptoms for millennia is changing, and there has been a slow-cooked emergence of hard research shining a spotlight on women navigating the time period that includes both perimenopause and menopause. Because of that, we are discovering the extent to which menopause causes system-wide changes in women, and particularly, for purposes of this book, how we can best influence our immune system and the gut microbiome to improve our overall health during this time and, really, for the rest of our lives.

What is the difference between perimenopause and menopause, exactly? Perimenopause is the time when a woman's body starts getting ready for **menopause**, which is when she stops having her period completely. It usually happens over a five- to ten-year period starting when a woman is in her late thirties or early forties. Perimenopause is the transition time before menopause, when the body slowly adjusts to having lower levels of certain hormones (especially progesterone and estrogen). Because so much information in this book spans both perimenopause and menopause, however, I use the umbrella term *middlepause* throughout the book.

Besides changes to our metabolism, sleep, and mental acuity, the decrease in estrogen and other reproductive hormones that comes with "the change" also wreaks havoc on our immune system, and we simply become more susceptible to opportunistic infections and other inflammatory issues. And where does the bulk of our immune system reside? In our gut. The composition of our gut microbiome shifts over the course of our lifetime and is at its most diverse in our late twenties and early thirties and starts to change in our midforties. This is when our microbiome is, typically, at its healthiest. The impact of the loss of sex hormones on the gut microbiome is substantial; research indicates that menopausal women have lower microbial diversity, changes in microbial richness, low-grade inflammation, and bacterial translocation (when bacteria cross our gut lining and enter areas where they do not belong—lymph, bloodstream, etc.). These changes impact metabolism, inflammation, mood, cognition, and bone health.

Here comes the one-two punch. The changes in my hormones and thus my immune system not only primed me to be much more susceptible to these opportunistic infections but also made it increasingly difficult to fight them off. With the decline of estrogen in my gut, my symptoms were exacerbated as my immune system became under-responsive and more impacted by exposure to pathogens. I had never put all these pieces together until now.

The gastrointestinal tract presents the largest surface and is most vulnerable to the outside world. It must simultaneously be accessible to nutrients and defend against pathogens and toxins. And menopause messes with these otherwise fierce defensive capabilities. That explained how my husband had eaten the same food and had no problems, while I got violently sick, and even afterward, it kept my body in a hyperaware state.

Stay with me, this isn't all bad news. Because research suggests a bidirectional relationship between our sex hormones and the gut microbiome—that is, higher levels of estrogen and progesterone promote increased microbial diversity and help maintain the integrity of the gut barrier (among many other benefits)—there is a path forward to helping build back the gut and maintain its integrity as we age. While the path isn't one-size-fits-all, it will guide you on finding what works for you, because until the medical community and research catch up, you have to educate yourself so you can be the best advocate for your own health.

That path is what you are now holding in your hands. This book will offer you evidence-based solutions I have found successful not only as my own guinea pig but also with hundreds of women within my clinical practice. I will first provide all the information you need about how systems work with our gut and how all that changes with perimenopause and menopause. I will then lay out a multitiered plan to help rebuild the gut for life after menopause—because, believe me, there is a good life to be had after menopause. By concentrating on lifestyle changes—such as nutrient density, meal frequency, your intake of fiber, adding ferments and prebiotics, sleep quality, exercise, and perhaps HRT and targeted supplementation—you will be able to build up a healthy postmenopausal immune system that should keep your body and mind running smoothly for life.

As I revisited this terrible health crisis when writing this introduction, I clearly saw there was the Cynthia before September 2018 and the Cynthia after. What I went through in 2018 and 2019 prepped me for the conversations that we're going to have within these pages, which will give you hard-won and well-researched information and advice you won't get from other doctors or practitioners. While many women face challenges in getting their symptoms recognized and treated by licensed healthcare providers, menopause doesn't have to be a life sentence. We don't have to suffer in silence. Informed means empowered. Armed with the knowledge that follows in this book—and other books by other women who are leading the change in menopausal health—you will be able to make better choices and achieve a greater awareness about how we can take our health to the next level. Because to me, it's about not just surviving but *thriving* through menopause. How about you?

The Menopause Gut

Part 1

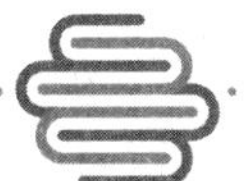

It's All Connected

Chapter 1

Getting to Know Your Microbiome

Menopause and perimenopause feel like crazy town. Just ask Melody. She is your type-A, do-it-all, I'll-sleep-when-I'm-dead kind of person. She was a star track athlete in college, and that dedication turned into running marathons. She used to run multiple marathons and even ran a few Iron-man competitions. She got by for years with four to five hours of sleep a night, often staying up late trying to catch up on work emails. She gave herself time to socialize but limited herself to five or six drinks a week, especially if she was stressed about her job as a graphic designer. But we all know that how we live in our twenties and thirties is not how we can live in our forties. And when she hit that milestone, she noticed she couldn't either, and the most significant change she saw was on the scale. While she never had to worry about how her clothes fit before, her pants were suddenly tight and she felt bloated all the time, so she was uncom-fortable in anything other than sweats or loose clothing. She didn't know she was hitting perimenopause, so, like many of us do, she started a diet. It was a time when fasting was becoming all the rage, so she tried it—specifically, OMAD (one meal a day). When that didn't do the trick, she came to see me.

We all know that bloated feeling. Your stomach feels so tight that it could burst, and your stomach growls, gurgles, and grumbles—sounds we would rather not have other people hear. It's just plain uncomfortable. Often, it can just be something we ate (or think we ate, like I thought in Morocco). But if you continue to have symptoms, it can be an indicator that something more nefarious is going on in your gut. As with many other functions in our body, we don't know something is wrong . . . until something is wrong. When our immune system is firing at full speed, it quietly but gallantly fights off bad bacteria while giving good bacteria a pass. But at times, that immune system stops working efficiently, and the cause is often the loss of equilibrium in our microbiome. And perimenopause and menopause are big factors in that equilibrium loss.

First things first. When I started practicing as an NP twenty years ago, the word *microbiome* had not been officially defined; it has been only in the past five to ten years that research has come out about how this microenvironment coexisting in your body is more than a mere plot of a science-fiction movie. What is it, exactly? Well, for one, it is "they." Trillions of they: The microbiome is really a catchall of the fascinating world of bacteria, fungi, viruses, and archaea that live mostly in your gut but also on your skin and in other parts of your body. It used to be thought that these tiny pathogens were bad, but we now know they can do a lot of good for us; in fact, we need them as much as they need us. Over the years, the medical community's understanding of the role of these microbes has expanded enormously, leading practitioners to discover their profound impacts on not only our digestion and metabolism but also our immunity, mental health, bone health, hormonal balance, and more.

The most studied microbiome is the gut microbiome—all twenty-five meters of it!—but microbiomes exist on the skin and in the mouth, vagina, and other areas of your body. For the purposes of this book, we'll concentrate on the gut microbiome and its bidirectional relationship with numerous other organ systems, including our brains, which help regulate a variety of processes, as well as our immune and nervous systems. In fact, according to *The British Medical Journal*, the microbiome should be considered a "virtual organ of the body" due to all these critical functions. It mainly lives in our gastrointestinal tract, particularly in the intestines, and the majority of microbes are found in the large intestine (also called the colon).

Throughout the GI tract is an intestinal layer, the epithelium, which lines the surface of the intestines—in some places only ten to fifty micrometers thick!—and serves as a crucial barrier between the gut contents and the rest of the body, while also playing a critical role in absorbing nutrients and interacting with the gut microbiome. It produces mucus, which allows the absorption of nutrients and fluids while acting as an efficient and protective barrier against toxins and microorganisms. Research has shown that the composition of the gut microbiome can vary significantly from person to person, but generally, there are six abundantly found bacteria in all of us: firmicutes, bacteroidetes, actinobacteria, proteobacteria, fusobacteria, and verrucomicrobia, among which firmicutes and bacteroidetes represent 90 percent of gut microbiota. Bacteroidetes are known for their ability to break down complex carbohydrates, while firmicutes are involved in the production of short-chain fatty acids (SCFAs), and actinobacteria help with the production of important digestive enzymes, all of which are important for gut health.

In Melody's case, her gut microbiome was taking a hit because of higher-than-normal estrogen levels, which is common in her grossly outdated nomenclature's "stage of life." Estrogen levels are typically 20 to 30 percent higher than during perimenopause and fluctuate more widely. What happens then? Well, we will get more into immunity in the next chapter, but in this case, high levels of estrogen increase our levels of histamine, a protein that is released by white blood cells in response to a stimulus (such as food) and acts as a defensive mechanism. We often see high estrogen levels (like in perimenopause) with high histamine levels, which can create a vicious cycle. (Dairy is a very common food sensitivity in perimenopause and menopause; it can be more inflammatory at this stage of life due to sensitivities or intolerances to key milk proteins like casein and whey, which can show up as gas, bloating, hives, eczema, nausea, or diarrhea.) Let's look a little bit into this relationship.

What a Healthy Microbiome Looks Like

This symbiotic relationship between our gut and its inhabitants dates back thousands of years. As our ancestors developed, these microbes adapted to live within us harmoniously. Studies suggest that our microbiomes have coevolved with us, influencing various aspects of our biology, immunity, and even behavior over time. A healthy microbiome comprises a wildly diverse microbial makeup, with bacteria being the most dominant, and the first time the body gets exposure to all these wonderful flora is most likely when we are born.

Before birth, the digestive tract is completely sterile, but it is then colonized immediately by the organisms we come into contact with. We acquire our first set of microbes from our mother during the birthing process. It's like getting our own private army of bacteria, protozoa, fungi, and viruses, which will form a protective barrier between the external environment and our internal environment. Many factors impact newborn microbiomes, including method of delivery (babies born vaginally tend to be more diverse than babies born via cesarean section), contact with parents, formula versus breastfeeding, and more, but it is a beautiful thing to see how our body intrinsically knows to protect itself. It's a rough world out here, and our body readies itself for a lifetime of battle. The period during your earliest development, especially within the first six months of life, is a critical time window for your microbiota—much change takes place. In the first few years of our lives, a genetic "imprinting" occurs in our gut microbiomes and thus determines the state of health moving forward. Even more than that, it can determine how we well we age.

Digestion and the Gut

Let's talk about the gut's main job: to break down what you eat, absorb all the nutrients, get rid of all the bad stuff, and ultimately provide energy throughout the body. It's a tall order, but when everything is working smoothly, the job gets done without you even knowing.

Your microbiome helps break down carbohydrates, proteins, fats, and other compounds that human enzymes can't digest on their own. How does it do that, exactly? A few ways. Most important, the gut bacteria break down the dietary fibers we eat into short-chain fatty acids like acetate, propionate, and butyrate. These in turn provide energy for our bodies, especially for the cells in our gut. They also keep inflammation at bay by inhibiting the production of pro-inflammatory cytokines and promoting the production of regulatory T cells (Tregs), which help suppress overactive immune responses. This is beneficial in preventing chronic inflammatory conditions like inflammatory bowel disease (IBD) and other gut-related disorders. SCFAs also help stabilize our metabolism by enhancing insulin secretion and modulating the release of gut hormones such as GLP-1 (glucagon-like peptide), regulating blood sugar levels by improving insulin (a hormone that helps control blood sugar), and reducing the risk of metabolic disorders like obesity and type 2 diabetes. If you remember the names of any of these, it should be butyrate. It is one of the most consequential, as it makes the lining of our gut stronger by tightening up the spaces between cells. This way, it stops harmful stuff from leaking into the bloodstream and triggering inflammation.

A healthy microbiome does a lot more than just help with digestion. Some gut bacteria produce crucial vitamins, like vitamin K, which is needed for our blood to clot and best absorb minerals like calcium (important for maintaining strong bones) and magnesium (important for muscles and nerves). They also help make B vitamins that give us energy, help build DNA, and keep our brains healthy. In addition, the microbiome helps break down bile acids in our body, which are needed to digest fats. This helps us absorb fats properly when we eat things like avocado, butter, and olive oil.

Your Immune System and Your Gut

The gut's second but no less important job is fortressing your immune system—in both its development and regulation. It's a big job—after all, 70 to 80 percent of your body's immune cells are in the gut. Gut microbes help train the immune system to distinguish between good substances (like nutrients we need for our bodies to function) and harmful viruses and other foreign invaders, keeping you safe and healthy.

A diverse microbiome helps prevent the overgrowth of bad bacteria. Basically, the more diverse your gut, the better your immune response. The strength of your immune system relies on the strength of the lining of the small intestine, which is structured to maximize nutrient absorption and is composed of several layers. It's important to understand how delicate this ecosystem is, so we'll dedicate the next chapter to this, but the crucial point is that if any of these areas are damaged or compromised, we will become susceptible to leaky gut—meaning food particles, bad bacteria, and other bad guys will leak into our bloodstream, leading to chronic inflammation.

That breach can lead to a leaky gut (increased small intestinal permeability), in which the lining of the small intestine becomes compromised, allowing substances like toxins, undigested food particles, and microbes to pass through the intestinal wall into the bloodstream. Normally, tight junctions between intestinal cells regulate what can pass through the gut lining. However, in leaky gut, these tight junctions loosen due to various factors such as stress, poor diet, infection, and overuse of medications like antibiotics, oral contraceptives, and nonsteroidal anti-inflammatory drugs (NSAIDs). This breach can activate the immune system, triggering chronic inflammation and contributing to autoimmune diseases such as celiac disease, Hashimoto's thyroiditis, rheumatoid arthritis, irritable bowel syndrome (IBS), and inflammatory bowel disease; this can be akin to inflammaging (a fancy term for chronic low-grade inflammation that occurs during the aging process).

The Gut and the Brain

Research shows the strong connection between the gut and the brain, what has been called the gut–brain axis: a bidirectional communication system that includes the nervous system, immune system, and hormones.

Do you know the phrase "trust your gut"? There is a lot of truth to that because this complicated information highway is so vital to our health and emotional well-being: The gut produces more than 90 percent of the body's neurotransmitters, including:

- **Serotonin**, which is widely known for its role in mood regulation, but it also plays a crucial role in regulating gut function, including bowel movements and peristalsis (intestinal muscle contractions). It also helps speed up digestion to get rid of toxic products or foods that irritate the body and can suppress appetite. Approximately 90 to 95 percent of the body's serotonin is produced in the gut, particularly by cells in the gut lining. Low serotonin can contribute to mood changes, anxiety, and depression, and can show up in our system as irritable bowel syndrome (IBS) or constipation.
- **Gamma-aminobutyric acid (GABA)**, which aids in our brain function and emotional states. Best known for its role in the central nervous system (our "second brain"), it functions as the primary neurotransmitter, helping regulate mood and stress levels. However, GABA also plays important roles in the gut, where it contributes to gut motility (the movement of food through the digestive tract), secretion, and sensation. Because GABA is involved in stress regulation, disruptions in its signaling can exacerbate stress-induced gastrointestinal issues. (This is why so many people complain about stomach issues when they are stressed.)
- **Dopamine**, a neurotransmitter best known for its role in the brain, where it regulates mood, motivation, reward, and motor control. However, dopamine also plays an important role in gut health. The gut microbiota can influence dopamine levels, affecting mood and behavior. Conversely, dopamine signaling from the brain can influence gut function, contributing to the regulation of gut motility and secretion. Dopamine dysregulation can trigger gastrointestinal disorders like IBS, and because dopamine is involved in regulating stress and reward pathways, changes in dopamine levels can exacerbate stress-induced gastrointestinal issues.

The microbiome also affects the production of hormones involved in appetite regulation, like leptin and ghrelin, thereby influencing energy balance and metabolic health. These hormones are part of the gut–brain axis, and their signaling can be influenced by the state of the gut microbiome, inflammation, and overall digestive health. In short, your microbiome is essential for digestion, immune function, metabolism, hormonal balance, mental health, and protection against disease. Thus, maintaining a healthy microbiome is *critical* for overall health.

Don't Forget to Set the Biological Clock

Another remarkable mechanism of our microbiome is that it helps our circadian clocks keep working, well, like clockwork. Our body operates on a twenty-four-hour clock, or circadian rhythm, and we have a master clock (a.k.a. a pacemaker) located in a small region of the hypothalamus called the suprachiasmatic nucleus (SCN), which is regulated by exposure to light as well as by mealtimes, life stages, and physical activities. There are clock cells—like tiny timers—throughout your body that work to control your internal clock, which helps regulate things like:

- Feeling sleepy or alert
- Hunger
- Body temperature
- Hormone production (like estrogen)
- Menstrual cycle

In addition, every cell in our body has its own "clock" that works off that twenty-four-hour schedule; your body working like clockwork promotes the health of your digestive system, mood, sleep, bones, and even hormones. Why is this important when talking about the gut? Because the microbiome is also heavily influenced by our nutritional (and not so nutritional) choices, it can in turn affect peripheral clocks in the gut and thereby influence the gut epithelium (lining) and the microbiota. This bidirectional relationship between our inner clocks and the gut microbiome means that disruptions in one can have profound effects on the other. If this is working correctly, your digestion will be in sync with your eating and sleeping habits. For example, your clock helps control when certain gut bacteria are more active. Some bacteria might help with digestion more in the day, while others work at night. Because gut microbes follow a circadian pattern, they fluctuate in response to feeding times, light-dark cycles, and sleep-wake patterns. During the day, gut bacteria involved in digestion and nutrient metabolism are more active, aligning with food intake and digestion. Certain bacterial species may peak in activity during the feeding phase (daytime), while others thrive during the fasting phase (nighttime). At night, when the body is fasting and the digestive system slows down, the microbiome shifts toward bacteria that help repair the gut lining, modulate immune responses, and maintain metabolic balance.

Circadian misalignment (disruptions in the natural circadian rhythm) can happen with changes to our schedule, such as shift work, jet lag, irregular sleep schedules, stress, and poor eating habits. All such changes can disturb the gut microbiome, potentially resulting in gut dysbiosis, which has been associated with various health problems such as decreased microbial diversity; metabolic disorders like obesity, insulin resistance, and type 2 diabetes; and increased risk of chronic diseases such as IBD, cardiovascular disease, and autoimmune disorders. So, when considering overall gut health, not only do we have to think of the health of the microbiome, we need to factor in the health of that circadian rhythm as well.

For Melody, whom you met earlier, it was evident that her high-octane lifestyle and occupational stressors, mixed with reaching perimenopause, had activated a complex network of hormones known as the hypothalamic–pituitary–adrenal (HPA) axis and upset her natural circadian clock. This disruption was exacerbated by changes in her sex hormones, specifically estrogen and progesterone.

So, her mood, sleep, and metabolism were off. To help her, we had her prioritize getting sunlight in the morning and use blue-blocking glasses at night, as these can both support the regulation of cortisol and melatonin secretion. I got her to commit to twelve to thirteen hours of a more gentle form of fasting called digestive rest, instead of OMAD, and we had her eating protein prior to her workouts. I suggested she avoid alcohol, and we added in restorative forms of exercise like yin yoga and swimming to give her body a rest from the constant high-level stress of long-form endurance and cardiovascular exercise. I also recommended progesterone, low-dose melatonin, and some adaptogenic herbs to help support sleep. Within a few months, she was back into her favorite jeans and was feeling more rested and less stressed.

What an Unhealthy Microbiome Looks Like

This fragile ecosystem is delicate, and when it becomes compromised, it reduces our ability to protect the digestive tract from pathogens that irritate our cells and create inflammation, diminishing our body's immunity.

There are many factors that contribute to disrupting this fragile environment, or what we call microbiome disruption or dysbiosis. We just learned that our circadian rhythm and our gut health are closely connected. But studies show that the American gut microbiome is less healthy than that of non-Western cultures. The culprit? Our overprocessed, nutrient-deficient diet. All this can lead to chronic inflammation, contributing to conditions like inflammatory bowel disease and other autoimmune diseases, allergies, asthma, type 2 diabetes, and certain cancers. Dr. William Davis discusses the role of lack of food diversity; food additives, like polysorbate 80 and carrageenan, negatively impacting the gut microbiome; heavy metals such as cadmium; the impact of BPA (bisphenol A); and the overuse of antibiotics, NSAIDs, proton pump inhibitors (stomach-acid-blocking drugs that are overprescribed), and statins (cholesterol medications). Some liken this to weeds in an otherwise beautiful garden. We're a motley crew of overexposure to items that profoundly damage our microbiome.

This dysbiosis is characterized by an imbalance in the composition, diversity, or function of the microbial community in the gastrointestinal tract. The imbalance can disrupt normal gut function, affect digestion, and contribute to a wide range of health issues. Several factors can lead to an unhealthy gut microbiome, and specific signs and characteristics can help identify this state.

Don't worry, though—dysbiosis can be alleviated with the right diet and lifestyle changes. Julia, age forty-six, was perimenopausal when she noticed an increase in her hot flashes as well as weight gain and fatigue. She felt depressed and anxious and had less energy for her day-to-day responsibilities. I ran some tests, which showed she had dysbiosis, low beneficial bacteria, low SCFAs (specifically butyrate), and high cortisol, suggesting late perimenopause and acute stress. To help support her, we increased her fiber intake slowly, as well as probiotic-rich foods; had her eliminate gluten entirely; added oral progesterone; and suggested breathwork/meditation and gentle yoga. She was feeling significantly better in six weeks.

Reduced microbial diversity: Reduced diversity is often linked to the Standard American Diet (SAD), excessive antibiotic use, chronic stress, and poor metabolic health. A lack of microbial variety can impair digestion, immunity, and the production of vital compounds like short-chain fatty acids. Decreased levels of beneficial bacteria, such as species of lactobacillus, bifidobacterium, and akkermansia, due to poor diet, stress, antibiotic use, or illness, can lead to impaired digestion, increased gut permeability (leaky gut), nutrient malabsorption, chronic inflammation, and conditions like IBS, obesity, and autoimmune diseases.

KEYSTONE BACTERIA

In the gut microbiome, **keystone bacteria** are VIPs that are especially important for keeping the gut healthy. While they aren't the most common bacteria in our gut and are super hard to pronounce, they have a huge influence, ensuring the whole community of bacteria in our gut works well together and thus making sure everything runs like a well-oiled machine. A few of their roles:

- **Produce helpful compounds:** Keystone bacteria like *Faecalibacterium prausnitzii* make substances like butyrate, a type of short-chain fatty acid, important to our gut health.
- **Support other good bacteria:** These bacteria create an environment where other helpful bacteria can grow. They're like the administrative arm of the gut, helping to make sure that good bacteria have what they need to thrive.
- **Protect against bad bacteria:** By keeping the gut environment healthy, keystone bacteria make it harder for harmful bacteria to take over. This helps prevent infections and keeps the immune system balanced.

Akkermansia muciniphilia, in short, helps maintain the gut lining. This bacterium is receiving a great deal of attention as new research has shown many potential benefits, such as support with endogenous GLP-1 production (which helps control appetite and slows digestion), its influence on SCFA production, and more. It's particularly important for gut health, as it helps production of mucus in the small intestine, which helps maintain the integrity of the gut lining and prevent the development of leaky gut syndrome. This species has also been shown to have anti-inflammatory properties and promote the production of key metabolites, such as butyrate, which are essential for gut health. Those with healthy levels are at lower risk for obesity, diabetes, and other chronic metabolic health conditions. Low levels of akkermansia are linked to metabolic disorders.

Faecalibacterium prausnitzii is another keystone species that has been shown to play a critical role in maintaining gut health, by producing anti-inflammatory compounds and promoting the growth of other beneficial bacteria in the gut. It also produces butyrate, which serves as an energy source for colon cells and has anti-inflammatory properties to keep the gut lining strong. It's one of the most abundant bacteria in healthy people, making up about 5 to 15 percent of the total gut microbiome. Low levels have been linked to IBD, Crohn's, ulcerative colitis, and other GI disorders.

Bacteroides fragilis helps maintain the balance of the gut ecosystem by regulating the immune response and producing important metabolites, such as short-chain fatty acids, that are essential for gut health. It produces PSA (polysaccharide A), which promotes a healthy immune system by better controlling inflammation. It plays an important role in T-cell responses, which in turn prevent inflammatory diseases and infections. So low levels or absence of *B. fragilis* can play a role in those inflammatory bowel diseases like Crohn's and ulcerative colitis, as well as in leaky gut and even colorectal cancer.

Lactobacillus species, particularly *Lactobacillus reuteri* and *rhamnosus*, produce lactic acid, which lowers the gut's pH level and inhibits the growth of harmful pathogens. These bacteria are also known for their probiotic properties, enhancing gut health by promoting beneficial microbes, reducing small intestinal hyper-permeability, and supporting a healthy immune response.

Bifidobacterium species are another important group of bacteria that promote a healthy gut environment, by fermenting dietary fibers and producing SCFAs like acetate, which supports the integrity of that oh-so-tiny small intestinal lining. These bacteria are especially important in infants because of their high nutritional needs as they grow and develop. They continue to support healthy digestion and immune system modulation throughout adulthood; low levels are linked to GI issues and metabolic disorders.

All this is to say that these keystone bacteria are critical in keeping your gut and immune system in check. If there aren't enough of them in the gut, it can lead to problems like digestive issues and may lead to diseases like IBD, in which the gut becomes irritated and inflamed. These VIP bacteria are essential for the proper functioning of the gut ecosystem, helping to break down food, produce important nutrients, and regulate the immune response—so it is important to get familiar with them. After all, they are living with you!

Overgrowth of harmful bacteria: Harmful bacteria can outcompete beneficial microbes, resulting in increased levels of toxins and inflammatory compounds that damage the gut lining and disrupt normal gut function. *Clostridium difficile* (*C. difficile*), *Escherichia coli* (*E. coli*), *Staphylococcus aureus*, and candida are examples of bacteria that can overgrow and cause inflammation and other digestive issues. Additionally, alterations in the small intestine can lead to overgrowth of bacteria (SIBO) or fungi (SIFO). When harmful bacteria proliferate or the gut lining is damaged, it can lead to increased gut permeability (leaky gut), allowing toxins, microbes, and undigested food particles to enter the bloodstream and trigger systemic inflammation. It is also linked to metabolic diseases, including diabetes, autoimmune diseases, food intolerances, and other inflammatory conditions.

What are the signs of a disrupted gut microbiome?

- **Digestive problems:** Bloating, gas, constipation, diarrhea, indigestion, and IBS-like symptoms are common signs of gut dysbiosis.
- **Food intolerances or sensitivities:** A lack of diversity in gut bacteria can impair the digestion of certain foods, leading to intolerances.
- **Chronic fatigue:** Dysbiosis can impact the gut–brain axis, contributing to fatigue and brain fog.
- **Mood disorders:** The gut microbiome influences mental health through the gut–brain axis. An unhealthy gut can contribute to anxiety, depression, and stress.
- **Skin conditions:** Due to the gut–skin axis, gut dysbiosis can be linked to skin issues like acne, eczema, and rosacea.
- **Frequent infections:** A weakened immune system, resulting from dysbiosis, can lead to recurring infections or illnesses.
- **Weight gain or weight-loss resistance:** This is the most common sign.

In addition, the gut microbiome plays a critical role in immune system regulation, helping to balance immune responses and protect against infections. An unhealthy microbiome can impair this function, leading to an overactive or weakened immune system. This can result in increased susceptibility to infections, higher rates of autoimmune diseases, and chronic inflammatory conditions.

Weight Gain / Weight-Loss Resistance

The changes in the gut microbiome associated with low estrogen, as well as other alterations in sex hormones, can influence metabolic health profoundly. In addition to this, we become less stress-resilient as we age, which potentially leads to weight gain or weight-loss resistance (WLR) and insulin resistance. These effects are significant because they contribute to the increased risk of metabolic syndrome, high blood pressure, polycystic ovarian syndrome (PCOS), diabetes, Alzheimer's, and more. Weight gain and WLR is a tough subject because so many variables contribute, such as:

- **Poor-quality sleep:** Getting less than seven to eight hours of sleep a night (like Melody) dysregulates the key hormones glucose, cortisol, and insulin, as well as the main hunger hormones (leptin and ghrelin), and will leave you without the benefits of restorative sleep. You will start craving foods that will not support a healthy lifestyle.
- **Stress:** Once we start transitioning from perimenopause into menopause, we have to be more proactive, as we steadily become less stress-resilient. This is a by-product of fluctuating levels of progesterone, which is one of the key sex hormones and has a wonderful antianxiety effect in the body. One of the hallmarks of early perimenopause is a reduction in secretion of progesterone by our ovaries. Our wonderful adrenal glands step in, like a backup quarterback, to help support our additional progesterone needs, but this further adds to our hindered ability to deal with chronic stress. Our adrenal glands are designed to be an emergency backup system, so in middle age, if we are not proactively managing our stress, our adrenals can get depleted. We have to go out of our way to decompress and put less stress on our bodies. Things as simple as

learning the value of saying no, meditation, or gentle yoga can go a long way at this stage of life in calming our autonomic nervous system. Most women spend their entire lives rushing from one thing to another, checking off their proverbial to-do list without realizing the harm they are causing long term. (We have an entire chapter devoted to stress later on in the book.)

- **Meal frequency:** Most Americans just eat too much and too frequently. Sugary coffee drinks, snacks, and mini-meals are all problematic in middle age. It *all* adds up. Learning to properly structure your meals with protein, healthy carbs, and fats is key, and if you can tolerate twelve hours of digestive rest or even intermittent fasting, great; there are so many benefits to eating less often.
- **Inflammatory or nutrient-deficient foods:** I gave up gluten at age forty and dairy at forty-five and never looked back. Both no longer worked for me. Many women do best with a lower-inflammation diet that is focused on nutrient-dense, less-processed foods and avoiding alcohol (sorry, my fellow wine lovers).
- **Protein:** We should be aiming for ideally a hundred grams a day of protein. If we don't eat sufficient protein, we will be left craving fat and carbs to make up for the caloric deficit. This is called the "protein leverage hypothesis." Everyone is different, of course, due to their own bio-individual needs, but changes in our diet can be critically impactful.
- **Toxins:** Between personal-care products, environment, and food, the average woman is exposed to hundreds of chemicals daily just with normal routines. Educate yourself and determine ways to reduce your exposure to toxins in your day-to-day life. Simple things like filtering your water, reading food labels, and avoiding the Environmental Working Group's Dirty Dozen go a long way toward this goal (see section on this very topic on page 121 to get started).
- **Hormonal shifts:** The fluctuating hormones that occur during perimenopause and menopause can wreak havoc on our changing

bodies. Shifts in progesterone, estrogen, and testosterone in particular can leave us feeling disconnected from ourselves and wondering where our old bodies went.

What Do Sex Hormones Have to Do with It?

As with most things—cars, cell phones, and yes, more "mature" bodies—age deteriorates performance and function. So why would we think anything different when it comes to the gut? And because hormonal balance is so closely linked to the microbiome, it should come as no surprise that as women age and go into perimenopause and menopause, there is a loss of microbial diversity.

But surprisingly, there hasn't been much research on this—until now. And while more research is still needed, we are seeing eye-popping connections between the depletion of sex hormones and the gut that we haven't seen before. We know, for instance, that perimenopausal and menopausal changes lead to a reduction in neurotransmitter production and the eventual decline in the sex hormone estrogen, which can impact the overall composition and function of the microbiome. With the decline in estrogen, predominantly estradiol (E2), women lose many protective effects on the gut microbiome and thus could see the following:

- **Shifts in microdiversity:** Estrogen receptors in the gut help regulate gut function and play a critical role in maintaining the diversity of the gut microbiome, meaning changes in levels of estrogen during middlepause will have a direct effect on diversity.
- **Increased risk of dysbiosis:** Gut microbiome changes during perimenopause and menopause can result in dysbiosis, a shift in the amount of beneficial bacteria versus bad bacteria, which can affect our immune and digestive functions as well as promote inflammation. In fact, less estrogen can contribute to overgrowth of non-beneficial bacteria, which further exacerbates leaky gut, inflammation, and potent toxins in the bloodstream called lipopolysaccharides (LPS). This is particularly important for women

navigating perimenopause and menopause, as lowered levels of ovarian hormones, like progesterone, influence mood and anxiety, sleep quality, and more. Translation: This is why you are tired and irritable!

- **Increased risk of inflammation:** The shift toward a less diverse microbiome can lead to a pro-inflammatory state, which is linked to various menopausal symptoms and long-term health risks, like cardiovascular disease, diabetes, and osteosarcopenia.
- **Decline in butyrate:** Postmenopausal changes in the gut microbiome are associated with a decline in butyrate (the SCFA that impacts gut-barrier integrity) and with inflammation and energy metabolism that may lead to leaky gut. We also see alterations in other SCFAs, like acetate and propionate, which may impact lipid metabolism and our appetites. In addition, the decline in estrogen can lead to an overall reduction in SCFA production, as less estrogen leads to fewer SCFAs, which can also lead to weight gain, insulin resistance, and more inflammation.
- **Digestive issues:** Lowered estrogen levels in middlepause often cause increased GI discomfort, including bloating, constipation, gas, flatulence, diarrhea, and IBS. These changes in the gut are potentially exacerbated by underlying food sensitivities and hormonal fluctuations.
- **Shifts in specific bacteria:** There's a tendency toward a decrease in beneficial bacteria, such as keystone bacteria lactobacillus and bifidobacterium, and an increase in potentially harmful bacteria, like enterobacterium. These changes contribute to GI symptoms commonly experienced in menopause, such as bloating and constipation.
- **Changes in metabolic function:** The gut microbiome's role in metabolizing nutrients and regulating energy balance can be compromised during menopause. This alteration may contribute to weight gain and changes in insulin sensitivity. Translation: This is one of many reasons you can't get rid of those five pounds as quickly as you used to.

We will talk more about the impact of estrogen on the microbiome in chapter 4, but for now, it is important to know that estrogen in the gut and the estrobolome—a subset of the gut microbiome responsible for metabolizing estrogen—decreases during menopause.

Restoring a Healthy Microbiome

So, what I've described isn't great news, but I promise there's hope! While these changes are inevitable as we age, there are many things we can do to stave off the worst effects of perimenopause and menopause and continue having a healthy and diverse microbiome. As with many health issues, if you fear your microbiome is out of whack, it can be improved by many of the resources we will discuss throughout this book, like the right diet (particularly unprocessed, fiber-rich, and probiotic-rich foods like yogurt, kimchi, and sauerkraut). Probiotics (beneficial live bacteria) and prebiotics (compounds that feed beneficial bacteria) can help restore microbiome balance. Eating the right amount of fiber and protein, especially SMASH fish (salmon, mackerel, anchovies, sardines, herring), polyphenol-rich fruits and veggies, and good sources of healthy fats (nuts, seeds, butter, olive oil, avocado), is a step in the right direction.

We will also get into hormone replacement therapy (HRT), including progesterone, estrogen, and testosterone, as other means of supporting our microbiome in perimenopause and menopause, as they can create protective effects in the gut. Exercise, better sleep, and stress management are also powerful tools, and we'll get into much more about what you can do in chapters 7–9.

Until then, now that you have a picture of the wonderfully lush world of the gut microbiome, let's explore how it interacts with our immune system.

Chapter Summary

1. The roller coaster of changes in estrogen levels during perimenopause and menopause greatly impacts the fragile environment of our microbiome. These changes can affect immune function, metabolism, inflammation, mood, cognition, bone health, and more—if we let it.
2. You may notice more anxiety, depression, or overall irritability at this time of life, which may impact how susceptible you are to opportunistic infections and autoimmune conditions.
3. Changes in sex hormones impact our central control clocks, which will in turn impact sleep quality, digestion, and more.
4. With lifestyle changes and good nutrition, you can keep your microbiome robust and plentiful.

References for this chapter can be found on my website: cynthiathurlow.com/themenopausegut-references

Chapter 2

Enemies at the Gate

At the age of forty-eight, Andrea, a busy grade-school teacher and mom of two, was not happy about the fact that her favorite foods weren't agreeing with her anymore.

"I noticed in the last few months, I have been having some uh, stomach issues when I had milk, cheese, or ice cream. I would feel nauseous and feel bloated. One time, I even got hives. What is up with this? Please don't tell me I can't have my favorite Cherry Garcia ice cream anymore."

"Are you still getting regular periods?" I asked her. It's always one of my first questions.

"Uh, well, yes, as of about five months ago, but it has been really spotty since then."

Andrea, like Melody, was in the throes of the later stages of perimenopause. Unfortunately, when perimenopause hits, changes occur in the microbiome, which in turn will affect our immune system. Andrea was becoming sensitive to dairy due to her fluctuating hormone levels, causing her to react more to foods like her beloved ice cream and cheese. The outcome: stomach upset and bloating, even though she never had a dairy allergy. That's why she was so perplexed when, all of a sudden, she couldn't tolerate her favorite foods.

Next to the brain, the immune system is the most complicated system of the body. While it is enormously complex, you don't need a medical degree to know this singular takeaway: Its main function is to keep out the bad stuff that can kill you or make you sick. And it is key to understand how it works, how the gut and immune system talk to each other, what happens when that communication goes awry, like during a time of stress and change—such as perimenopause and menopause—and most important, what we can do about it!

What Makes Up the Immune System?

While the immune system is incredibly intricate, involving your key organs like the lymph nodes (where cells train and communicate) and the spleen (which filters blood for unwanted guests), your skin, mucus, and stomach acid (barriers that keep invaders out before the fight even starts), I will keep this lesson limited to the immune system in the gut, as it holds about 70 to 80 percent of your immune cells, and there is intricate interplay between them and the intestinal microbiota. In addition to the local immune responses in the gut, it is increasingly recognized that the gut microbiome also affects our systems throughout the body. There's a saying, "What goes on in the gut does not stay in the gut." It is complicated, but I want you to think of this part of the immune system as an elite, around-the-clock army protecting your entire body from harmful invaders, but instead of warring countries, we are talking about unwanted bacteria, viruses, and other bad agents. This defense system involves multiple systems, much like different branches of the military—all working together to keep you healthy. (Until perimenopause and menopause, that is, when, in the wake of middle age, it all changes.)

At the forefront are white blood cells, on patrol, hunting down threats. Some, like macrophages, "eat" invaders, while others, like T cells, launch targeted attacks (think SEAL Team Six). Supporting them are B cells, which produce antibodies—custom weapons tailored to fight off specific enemies.

There are three places in the gastrointestinal (GI) tract where foods need to bypass these patrol cells and pass inspection: the intestinal microbiota, the intestinal epithelial layer, and the mucosa. The gastrointestinal wall of the GI is made up of four layers of tissue, but we want to concentrate on the innermost layer, called the mucosa, that surrounds the lumen of the tract and comes into direct contact with digested food. It has an essential role in digestion, nutrient absorption, and immune defense. There are three types of cells in this layer that are very important for getting what we need from food while kicking the bad stuff out: enterocytes, which are responsible for nutrient absorption; goblet cells, which produce mucus to protect and lubricate the lining; and dendritic cells (DCs), which serve as gatekeepers by constantly monitoring for pathogens.

Double Duty: Adaptive and Innate Immunity

Your delicate immune system keeps you safe—most of the time. A human consumes more than six million tiny microbes in and on our food every day—that is a huge workload for your immune system, and sometimes things can go awry (like with Andrea's new food sensitivities) or attack your own body (which occurs in any autoimmune disease). But to stave off any major crisis, the immune system employs two main defensive branches that work in tandem. They are two different but complementary divisions of labor: innate and adaptive immunity. You are born with your innate system. Being your first line of defense, it reacts quickly to invaders and in a somewhat haphazard way, but it gets the job done. It's in active mode 24-7, so it is ready whenever a foreign entity enters the body. It recognizes all types of pathogens, including bacteria, fungi, and viruses. Think of your white blood cells as the body's first responder, those foot soldiers on the front lines, providing a quick and broad defense that kicks in as soon as trouble starts (such as a fever or a sore throat—that's the immune system trying to fight off the virus causing the cold).

Adaptive immunity takes longer to develop because it evolves from learned experiences. Think of it as the higher-ups in the military—the generals and leaders who create tactical and strategic decisions based on what they've learned from past battles and build a memory, meaning the next time you encounter the same enemy, your body strikes faster and harder. It keeps a record of every potential pathogen you've encountered, so that it can recognize and destroy it when it enters your body again, utilizing more precise weaponry that targets the specific germ you're trying to fend off. It's slower to react but smarter: Once it fights off an infection, it remembers the invader, making future responses faster and stronger. (This more sophisticated type of immunity is what makes vaccines effective.) It's as if your own defense department made a playbook for future reference, and they update it each time they meet a new enemy.

This ready-made immune system's main line of defense is in the gut. This is crucial because the gut is exposed to a constant influx of foreign substances, including food, toxins, and microbes. How does it do this? Your gut is on constant surveillance, and it responds quickly, crudely, but effectively with these physical barriers (here the mucus layer), which trap pathogens like a spiderweb and protect the ecosystem from harm. Then those immune cells and gut go on high alert and they all respond in tandem and quickly, acting to avoid pathogen spread, but at the same time activating the adaptive immune system.

What does this look like? Your system could be triggered by something as simple as eating a highly processed food—say, a granola bar—that you bought at the local deli while you were out on errands. While it seems like a benign choice, this bar is like a pipe bomb going off in your gut. Most of its ingredients have been exposed to glyphosate, an herbicide and pesticide commonly found in our food supply, which can damage the small intestinal lining. It's all hands on deck as your immune cells come to the rescue to put the fire out, inevitably causing inflammation.

If our adaptive immunity is chronically activated, it can lead to inflammation and inflammaging that may show up as joint pain, fatigue, brain fog; a higher risk of developing autoimmune conditions; a greater chance of developing leaky gut, leading to food sensitivities; and issues in the gut–brain axis that can cause mood disorders such as depression and anxiety.

The Intricate World of the Innate Immune System

Your innate immunity is crucial because our bodies are exposed to a constant influx of foreign substances, including food, toxins, and microbes (both beneficial and harmful). It responds quickly and crudely but effectively in its physical barriers, like skin, stomach acid, and the gut's mucus layer, which contains immune cells that capture and kill off pathogens and protect our fragile ecosystem from harm.

The second line of defense—your adaptive immunity—relies on white blood cells that travel through the bloodstream and into tissues to literally swallow and destroy pathogens such as bacteria and dead cells in a process called phagocytosis. This is a crucial part of clearing infections and cleaning up cellular debris from damaged tissues.

Your innate immunity also relies on its dendritic cells throughout your body where there is contact with the external environment, like the skin (especially the epidermis) and the lining of the nose, lungs, and intestines. They serve as gatekeepers by constantly monitoring for pathogens and helping maintain tolerance to friendly gut bacteria and food. Consider these the liaison officer between your adaptive and innate immunity branches. They are responsible for capturing, processing, and presenting antigens (foreign molecules or pathogens) to T cells, thereby initiating and shaping the adaptive immune response. In women, estrogen enhances the antigen-presenting ability of dendritic cells, leading to more robust T-cell activation and a stronger overall immune response.

Adaptive Immunity

Let's dig deeper. Acquired immunity, also known as adaptive immunity, plays a vital role in protecting women from infections and diseases by providing a specific immune response based on prior exposure to pathogens. This slower-acting and more sophisticated system, in the form of white blood cells, is alerted by the innate immune system; these guys take a little more time in their attacks, as they are more specific and targeted. Much like an army's generals, they make plans according to what happened on the battlefield and create strategies for the future. They are measured, slow, but smart, while the innate system is the foot soldier—fast, quick acting, but more instinctual.

In women, acquired immunity is influenced by several factors, including hormones, genetics, and life stages such as pregnancy and menopause. These factors can lead to differences in immune responses, contributing to stronger pathogen defenses and a higher incidence of autoimmune diseases in women.

The gut microbiome works with your adaptive immunity, influencing its development and function. Beneficial microbes in the gut help train adaptive immune cells, specifically T cells (white blood cells that help recognize a threat) and B cells (white blood cells responsible for producing antibodies to that threat), to help your body recognize and attack germs or infected cells, but they are very specific—meaning each T cell can only recognize one specific threat. T cells help the body's overall tolerance and enhance its ability to mount targeted responses to infections. And even though short-chain fatty acids are not part of adaptive immunity, they affect how T cells and B cells develop and respond.

Sex Hormones Come into Play with Our Innate Immune System, Too

I told you the immune system is complicated. With all the immune cells I've described, you'd think we were all set in our defenses. Not yet—your sex hormones (chemical messengers) come into play as well. There has been remarkable new research on how the immune system differs by gender. In women, innate immunity tends to be more vigilant and robust compared with that of men. For example, we have discovered in recent years that estrogen, the main female sex hormone, broadly stimulates immune system activity. How is that, exactly? Well, it goes pretty deep into our DNA: Women have two X chromosomes, while men have one X and one Y chromosome. The X chromosome contains many genes related to immune function, including those that regulate pattern recognition receptors (PRRs), such as toll-like receptors (TLRs), which are important for detecting pathogens. Our double X chromosome gives us a genetic advantage in terms of immune system robustness, as we have a "backup" set of immune-related genes. This genetic redundancy allows for a more resilient and charged immune response, although this can also mean an increased susceptibility to autoimmune diseases due to possible overactive immune responses.

There have been clinical and animal studies that have demonstrated they can facilitate many of the gender-specific immune responses, from the susceptibility to infectious diseases to the prevalence of autoimmune disorders. Specifically, estrogen and progesterone have significant effects on innate immune function in women. These hormones fluctuate during the menstrual cycle, pregnancy, and menopause, and these fluctuations impact the immune system in different ways. Estrogen stimulates the immune system; progesterone tends to decrease the inflammatory response. Together, they typically work to balance each other out. Estrogen receptors, which house themselves in most immune cells, enhance the activity of each cell, which in turn improves their ability to detect and eliminate pathogens. Similarly to estrogen, there are progesterone receptors found on many different types of immune cells, including macrophages, B and T lymphocytes, and natural killer cells.

Let's take estrogen first: This hormone boosts the production of cytokines (messengers that communicate between cells to coordinate an immune response), chemokines, and reactive oxygen species (ROS), all of which contribute to the inflammatory response in infections. During perimenopause, women can experience high fluctuations of estrogen. As I mentioned in chapter 1, one of the ways this affects the body is by triggering the production of the chemical histamine through the immune system's mast cells, often in response to things it thinks are harmful, like certain foods or allergens. In women with high estrogen, the body might release too much histamine, leading to sensitivities to certain foods—like dairy—or even hives. This means that eating dairy during this time could cause uncomfortable symptoms, which can create a cycle in which high estrogen leads to high histamine, and high histamine causes more food sensitivities. So, in perimenopause, some women might notice they become more sensitive to foods like dairy because of this connection between estrogen and histamine. This is what happened to Andrea. Her body was in overdrive, releasing histamines and making her suddenly unable to enjoy her beloved ice cream.

Additionally, lower estrogen levels in menopause impact our ability to fight infections and increase inflammation and oxidative stressors. This is why women are more susceptible to urinary tract infections (UTIs) and vaginal infections in menopause, when our systemic estrogen levels are low. There's more to the changes in immunity in our genitourinary systems at middle age, including changes in the pH level that are brought on by less estrogen to feed the healthy lactobacillus and, overall, thinner vaginal epithelial tissue. Ouch!

Progesterone is a bit less understood but equally important as estrogen in regulating the immune responses. Progesterone rises during the luteal phase (days fifteen through twenty-eight) of the menstrual cycle, and during pregnancy, and has an immunosuppressive effect on innate immunity. Think of this hormone as a thermostat, helping modulate the immune system and adjusting it, based on our needs, to protect against excessive inflammation and prevent the immune system from attacking the developing fetus during pregnancy. All this gets impacted in perimenopause and menopause.

Progesterone decreases the activity of natural killer cells and the production of pro-inflammatory cytokines, which may explain why women are more susceptible to certain infections during the luteal phase of their cycles and during menopause. The hormone also reduces the production of cytokines, which are involved in promoting inflammation, and enhances cytokines, which support a more anti-inflammatory response. While I have found little research on testosterone, we do know that testosterone also has an immunosuppressive effect on our bodies; it actually suppresses a component of our adaptive immune response, namely our T cells. Most research on androgens (testosterone is one of several of this hormone class) centers around PCOS; the data suggests a correlation between the endocrine and immune systems. In PCOS, we know that there are specific changes to the microbiome that may impact microbial diversity and specific bacterial shifts.

Inflammatory Responses in Innate Immunity

Women tend to mount a more robust inflammatory response than men due to hormonal and genetic factors. From an evolutionary perspective, women may have developed their enhanced innate immunity as a protective mechanism, particularly during pregnancy and child-rearing, when the health of the mother is crucial for the survival of her children. The stronger immune responses in women may have provided an evolutionary advantage by helping them fend off infections during critical reproductive periods, ensuring better outcomes for both mothers and children.

While this heightened inflammatory response is essential for quickly eliminating infections, it also increases the risk of excessive inflammation and tissue damage. How? Estrogen enhances the production of pro-inflammatory cytokines, which are important for fighting infections.

However, excessive levels of these cytokines can contribute to chronic inflammation and inflammatory diseases. This helps explain why women are disproportionately more prone to autoimmune diseases—approximately 80 percent of all autoimmune cases occur in women. The same mechanisms that help women fight off infections more effectively may turn against the body's own tissues and lead to conditions like lupus, rheumatoid arthritis, and multiple sclerosis.

DARK AND STORMY

A **cytokine storm** happens when your body's immune system goes a little out of control. It's like an alarm system that doesn't stop ringing, even after the danger is gone. Normally, cytokines call for help when there's an infection, and when the job is done, they calm down and stop. In a cytokine storm, the immune system keeps sending out more and more cytokines, even if the infection is already under control. This makes the immune system overreact and attack not just the germs but also healthy cells in the body, causing a lot of inflammation (swelling and redness) throughout. It's like a small fire turning into a big, uncontrollable blaze that spreads everywhere. This can cause a variety of symptoms, much like having the flu, and can threaten important organs like the lungs, heart, and kidneys.

If there is one thing we can celebrate as women, it's the fact that we have a more vibrant immune response than men. Women generally produce stronger antibody responses to infections and vaccinations, which is a key aspect of acquired immunity. This enhanced response is often linked to estrogen, which modulates the activity of the immune system's B cells and supports higher antibody titers after vaccination or infection. While estrogen generally enhances innate immune activity, progesterone modulates it, especially during pregnancy, to prevent excessive inflammation. The balance between these hormones and the innate immune system is critical for women's health; however, while this heightened immune vigilance provides better protection against infections, it also raises the risk of chronic inflammatory and autoimmune conditions. In general, autoimmune disease (AD) develops when the innate and adaptive immune responses go awry. A combination of both genetics and environment contribute to the susceptibility to developing AD. Instead of just attacking the bad germs, the immune system gets confused and starts attacking healthy parts of our own body by mistake, like our skin, joints, or organs. This can cause damage and make us feel sick. Think of it like a fire alarm in a house. It's supposed to go off when there's a fire (a real threat), but in autoimmune diseases, the alarm keeps going off even when there's no fire. This causes problems and damages the house (our body).

In Andrea's case, her gut microbiome was taking a hit because of wildly fluctuating estrogen levels. Estrogen levels are typically 20 to 30 percent higher during perimenopause and fluctuate more widely. It's not just food sensitivities; you can also have breast tenderness, heavy menstrual cycles, weight-loss resistance, headaches, or even migraines. Out-of-balance estrogen can precipitate diagnoses like endometriosis, ovarian cysts, or even fibrocystic breasts. With less circulating estrogen, innate immune cells become easily over-activated via the first line of defense, which contributes to a cascade of effects, including systemic inflammation in the brain, bloodstream, heart, and everywhere else in the body.

And it's not just estrogen. Progesterone can play a big part in our suffering through menopause. If these two hormones are not balanced together, symptoms like bloating can occur. Low progesterone can show up as insomnia, anxiety, depression, and overall malaise.

How does this happen? Our bodies' T cells, another critical component of acquired immunity, are modulated by sex hormones like estrogen and progesterone. Estrogen enhances their responses, which in turn promote a stronger overall immune response. Progesterone helps buffer this response. Women suffer more from autoimmune diseases like systemic lupus erythematosus (SLE), Hashimoto's thyroiditis, rheumatoid arthritis, and multiple sclerosis. The same factors that strengthen pathogen defenses can also make the immune system more likely to attack the body's own skin, joints, and organs.

We also see significant shifts in perimenopause and menopause due to ovarian aging. For example, in perimenopause and especially in menopause, lower estrogen makes women more susceptible to urinary tract infections (changes in pH of the vaginal microbiome, shifts in beneficial bacteria of the urethra and vaginal vault). Additionally, other critical factors can impact estrogen levels, such as chronic stress, altered circadian rhythms (lack of sleep), and use of oral contraceptives; women have to be extra vigilant.

What Changes in Menopause?

In one sentence? Our immune system becomes less efficient and less effective. In lab studies, we see specific immune marker changes in menopause, like an increase in pro-inflammatory markers, a decrease in the number of those pathogen-fighting T and B cells, and a decrease in the cytotoxic activity of natural killer cells. How does this disruption translate into real life? Well, it's complicated because every woman's experience at this stage of life is as unique as she is. Estrogen can influence the function of immune cells in various tissues and organs, so some women may notice immune-related symptoms, such as an increase in infections, while others may observe shifts in preexisting autoimmune conditions, all due to chronic inflammation caused by a compromised immune system brought on by menopause. In my clinical experience, in perimenopause and menopause I see a great deal of hypothyroidism, an underactive thyroid that exhibits itself as weight gain, brain fog, dry skin and hair, constipation, fatigue, and inability to endure the cold; and Hashimoto's, an autoimmune disorder that affects the thyroid and can cause hypothyroidism. It starts as a "slow boil" in perimenopause and just gets more magnified as we navigate into our menopausal years. Increased levels of inflammation, over time, will deregulate and erode the immune response and our ability to fight infection.

Approximately 90 percent of people diagnosed with hypothyroidism are impacted by Hashimoto's. One of them was Charlene, who came to me with significant fatigue, dry skin, "terrible" constipation, hair loss, and irregular cycles. I strongly suspected that her thyroid was contributing to these symptoms. Her lab results showed low thyroid levels (T3 and T4) and high antibodies. Her serum magnesium, vitamin D, and selenium were low. Her progesterone was also low. We started compounded T3 and T4, and we added supplements to address her low magnesium, vitamin D, and selenium levels. We added progesterone in the second half of her cycle. I asked that she also commit to going gluten- and dairy-free. At her six-week appointment she told me she had less constipation, her dry skin had improved, and she didn't see as much hair circling the drain as she used to. Most important, she had more energy and was able to start going back to her favorite yoga class.

Tissue and joints: This change can cause microscopic damage to our tissues and impair our ability to repair and recover. For example, if someone in middlepause falls and sprains a wrist, it will take two times as long to recover. If that person has persistent low-level inflammation that shows up as joint swelling (edema), redness (erythema), or pain with movement (inflammation), that joint may take much longer to heal—or may never fully recover. One example of this: Adhesive capsulitis, a.k.a. frozen shoulder, is common in perimenopause and menopause. I have seen so many women get this and be utterly perplexed why, but it's related to reduced levels of estrogen and increased inflammation. It's even more common in women not taking HRT.

The microgenderome: This is a fancy word for the interaction between gut microbiome, sex hormones, and immune system. Recall that there's a bidirectional relationship between our gut microbiome and all systems in the body. And the differences between sexes can lead to changes in immunity, inflammation, and susceptibility to specific disease. So, what does that mean? An unhealthy gut microbiome can mean an unhealthy rest of the body. While this book focuses on the gut microbiome, we can see changes in all microbiomes (skin, vaginal, oral, respiratory), which make us likely to develop skin, vaginal, and urinary issues; dental and oral care issues and tooth loss; and lung infections, such as pneumonia and bronchitis. Additionally, changes in the innate immune system impact mucus membranes in the gut microbiome, and because the nose, throat, and vagina are the first line of defense to help keep pathogens out, colds, viruses, and the flu can be more problematic if the mucus membranes are weakened.

Our female parts: As a result of the loss of estrogen, there are structural changes in the lining of the vagina that impact the pH of the tissue and the bacterial species (healthy lactobacillus). The loss of this bacterial species leads to a reduction in mucus production, which then leads to a reduction in lubrication and gives us the dreaded dryness, itching (pruritus), and pain down there. These changes (called GSM, or genitourinary syndrome of menopause) can leave women more susceptible to not only micro-tears and painful sex but also opportunistic infections, like UTIs. An estimated 10 to 15 percent of women over sixty years of age suffer from frequent urinary tract infections. Chronic UTIs can be particularly annoying—I can't tell you how many of my middle-aged and older patients were on low-dose antibiotics for their recurring UTIs. (What they really needed was low-dose vaginal estrogen, but we'll get to that later in the book.) There is solid research that HPV (human papillomavirus) has a second peak prevalence in middle-aged women in the menopausal transition, and it is believed that the new HPV infections among older women are attributable to reduced immune responses. There is also research suggesting that menopausal females may be susceptible to HIV infections as well (although this increase may be attributed to not using protection because there is a zero chance of pregnancy).

Leaky gut and food sensitivities: Inflammation in the gut microbiome shows up as loss of diversity and an increased likelihood of developing dysbiosis and leaky gut. If the tight junctions are damaged, it allows undesirable items to pass directly into the bloodstream and exacerbate an immune response or help drive food sensitivities. This leakage into the bloodstream then creates both a localized and a systemic effect. It gets magnified. Andrea's new reaction to dairy is a great example of how our immune system and sex-hormone changes in perimenopause make us more susceptible to immunity issues; in her case, her new food sensitivities sparked unwanted bodily responses. For Andrea, high estrogen begets high histamine (a protein released by white blood cells in response to a stimulus, such as food). I saw it with her, and I see it with many women who develop reactions to milk, cheese, and other dairy products—something they'd tolerated their entire lives, and all of a sudden they became dairy intolerant, driving an inflammatory cascade in the body. This histamine response can occur with many types of foods, not just dairy; I've seen it with high-histamine healthy fermented foods, like kombucha, miso, and sauerkraut, as well as beans, nuts, and many others.

Inflammation markers: Chronic inflammation can show up in labs as well. A common marker is high-sensitivity C-reactive protein (hs-CRP), a protein made by the liver that increases when there's inflammation in the body, as well as metabolic health markers, like fasting insulin and glucose. This chronic inflammation puts menopausal women at greater risk of developing cardiovascular disease, which is the number one cause of death in women. Inflammation markers have also been recently shown to be important independent risk factors for cardiovascular disease in postmenopausal women. In one study, postmenopausal women were older, weighed more, and had greater total fat mass and intra-abdominal fat than premenopausal women. These changes to fat mass and lean body mass further exacerbate inflammation and shift our metabolic health in negative ways, specifically loss of muscle mass and increased insulin resistance.

What Comes Down: The Decline in Estrogen and Its Effect on Adaptive Immunity

Estrogen also plays a critical role in modulating the adaptive immune response. During the reproductive years, estrogen enhances the activity and proliferation of T and B cells, boosting the body's ability to fight infections and respond to vaccines. After menopause, the decline in estrogen results in less robust T cell responses and diminished antibody production from B cells, leading to a weakened adaptive immune response. What does that mean for you? You may get more frequent colds, recurring UTIs, thinner skin or hair, and autoimmune flares, as well as thyroid-related issues like weight gain, constipation, dry skin, and brain fog, which can all be signs of an underactive thyroid.

T cells, critical for recognizing and eliminating infected or cancerous cells, decline in functionality with age. In menopausal women, this decline is accelerated due to reduced estrogen levels. Specifically, cytotoxic T cells and helper T cells become less effective, which can lead to a higher susceptibility to viral infections and a decreased ability to fight cancer cells. Memory T cells, which "remember" past infections or vaccinations, may also decrease in number or function, leading to a weaker response to previously encountered pathogens.

Changes in Immunity with Aging

If we didn't have enough to worry about, menopause is not the only thing that chips away at our immune system. Immunosenescence—the gradual deterioration of the immune system brought on by the aging process—is another culprit. Immunosenescence brings with it a decrease in the response to pathogens and increased rates of morbidity and mortality. This, per se, does not mean that getting sick will bring the grim reaper knocking on your door; it simply means that our immune systems aren't as vibrant as they once were. The aging process leads to changes in both innate and adaptive immunity. It's also linked to inflammaging, characterized by chronic, low-grade inflammation that is associated with the aging process itself. Consequently, aging of the immune system results in an increased susceptibility to infections and decreased response to vaccination.

The immune system ages just like any other part of the body, and this leads to a decrease in its efficiency in fighting disease as it struggles more to distinguish between healthy cells and disease invaders. This decline is gradual but becomes more noticeable for women as they approach their menopausal years, and it can be hastened by chronic stress. The immune system's diminished ability to distinguish between harmful and benign cells may increase inflammation and susceptibility to infections, contributing to autoimmunity issues and tissue damage. Chronic low-grade inflammation contributes to a higher risk of age-related diseases like cancer, cardiovascular disease, diabetes, and osteoporosis. And here's an added complication: As studies show that we are living longer, women's post-menopausal timeline is no longer a stage that screams old age; it is fast becoming one third of their lives.

All this can be exacerbated by stress. I know: I had a few lingering but manageable inflammations spread like wildfire in my body. All of a sudden, I was exhausted, had trouble sleeping, and became weight-loss resistant. I had a sympathetic healthcare provider who performed extensive labs and listened intently to what I was experiencing; I knew my body well and it was not responding to my usual strategies (namely, exercise more + eat less = weight loss). It was evident that I had multiple variables at play, not the least of which was severe hypothyroidism. I needed thyroid replacement medication. Initially, I was very hesitant, not wanting to take medication for the rest of my life. However, after about six months, I finally relented. I felt better on medication within two to three days! Along with other lifestyle changes—better sleep habits, less intense gym workouts, and a more nutrient-dense diet—I was able to balance my immune system. (Yes, even we medical providers, who should know better, need help every so often.)

Don't Forget These Hormones That Impact Immunity

Many hormones impact our immune system (I told you it was complicated!), not just our sex hormones, and I will devote a later chapter to them. For now, keep in mind how the following can also be critical to our immunity:

DHEA is a hormone produced in the adrenal glands, above the kidneys. It's a precursor to male and female sex hormones, such as testosterone and estrogen, meaning it can become whichever hormone is needed at the time. It helps activate the immune system and plays an important role in modulating acute stress.

Cortisol is a hot topic these days, probably because everyone is worried about their stress levels. And we become less stress-resilient with age. What we tolerated in our twenties and thirties is no longer manageable, again due to hormonal fluctuations as our bodies prepare for the loss of fertility.

When our body functions normally, cortisol helps maintain our immune response. Typically, the body's reactions to a perceived threat—fight or flight—are in short spurts; our cortisol levels go up to respond to a threat and then return to normal after the threat is gone. But if that response becomes chronically high—whether it's a crisis at work, family discord, or health issues, we all seem to be battling a constant onslaught of stress—we remain in fight-or-flight mode. In that state, the immune system can become compromised, and our bodies become less adept at preventing infections, increasing the likelihood of developing autoimmune conditions and other diseases, such as cancer. Think: Short-term inflammation heals; long-term inflammation leads to disease. And guess what. Just like the rest of the hormones, cortisol does not get off scot-free from the effects of menopause. During this time, abnormal cortisol levels are common, which can compromise our immune system by decreasing antibodies, increasing inflammatory substances like cytokines, and reactivating latent viruses (hello, shingles, which is simply reactivation of the varicella virus after chickenpox!). Speaking of latent virus reactivation, did you know that the lifetime probability of shingles reactivation is estimated to be 10 to 30 percent, and the risk considerably increases to over 50 percent in patients age eighty-five and older? In case you forgot, our chickenpox experience as a kiddo can show up as shingles in an adult. Same virus (varicella), but more problematic with age. So, this is just another reason to protect your health by proactively managing stress in middle age.

STRESS, CORTISOL, AND ACEs

There is increasing evidence that trauma in childhood can greatly affect our immunity. Adverse childhood experiences (ACEs), such as abuse or neglect, can cause chronic over-activation of our sympathetic nervous system, which primes our bodies for an inability to downregulate our immune system after exposure to stressors. Over time, this over-activated system will cause cortisol dysregulation and lead to the body's debilitation. These immunological effects of chronic stress and elevated cortisol, especially starting at a young age, can advance cellular aging (immunosenescence) and shorten telomere length (which ages us faster!).

ACE stressors can also significantly impact women's health during menopause. A study by the Mayo Clinic found that women with a history of ACEs reported more severe hot flashes and night sweats during menopause. Additionally, these women experienced higher levels of psychological symptoms, including depression and anxiety. And a study published in the journal *Menopause* showed that women who experienced abuse from childhood through early adulthood had significantly worse general well-being and more challenging menopausal symptoms, such as sleep disturbances and sexual dysfunction.

We'll talk more about the long-term implications of ACEs in chapter 9.

Insulin is the hormone that helps regulate blood sugar, but it also affects the immune system in a few complicated ways. The big takeaway is that if your blood sugar is too high or too low, it can disrupt your body's immune response, making it harder to fight infection. Typically, estrogen keeps insulin sensitivity at a steady rate, but as menopause creeps in and estrogen levels decline, women become more susceptible to weight gain, poor metabolic health, and even type 2 diabetes.

The **thyroid** produces and secretes a number of hormones and helps regulate almost every organ in the body by helping them control how they use energy. Our metabolism, heart rate, and breathing are all monitored by hormones released by the thyroid. Here's where menopause comes into play: Researchers found that estrogen levels might affect thyroid function and lead to disorders of the gland. The bidirectional communication between the thyroid and the immune system is complex and not fully understood, but what we do know is that 12 to 20 percent of women over the age of sixty have an underactive thyroid, which happens when the immune system attacks the thyroid gland. What does that translate into? Weight gain, fatigue, and hot flashes.

Melatonin, everyone's favorite hormone, regulates your sleep cycle or your circadian rhythm. It is also a master antioxidant for the body. There are melatonin receptors throughout our bodies, including in the intestines, fat tissue, kidneys, lungs, adrenals, and other organs. We'll talk about the role of circadian rhythm and microbiome in chapter 4 in great detail, but for now, understand this comes into play with our immunity as well. Melatonin is a major regulator of the immune system and decreases with age, and less of this hormone equals—you guessed it—less quality sleep, more inflammation, and higher susceptibility to disease.

Tying It All Together

It never ceases to amaze me how the immune system works to keep us safe and yet can go awry so quickly. Because changes in our gut and hormones affect our immune system negatively, there is an uptick in so many issues as women hit their forties, fifties, and sixties. But it doesn't have to be this way. While none of us can avoid aging and menopause, we don't have to accept that this beautiful system becomes less effective as we age. We can do something to combat it, but before we get to how, let's find out how our ovaries also age.

Chapter Summary

1. The immune system is incredibly intricate, and the gut houses 70 to 80 percent of those important immune cells. So, you are what you eat.
2. A decline in immune function is the most recognized sign of aging.
3. Changes to the immune system are magnified by the loss of estrogen.
4. Inflammaging is chronic, low-grade inflammation associated with the aging process.

References for this chapter can be found on my website: cynthiathurlow.com/themenopausegut-references

Chapter 3

Ovaries Age, Too

One of the most telltale signs of postmenopause is simply no longer having a menstrual cycle. While some rejoice that they no longer need to have a steady stash of tampons, others see it as an emotional reminder that they are indeed not immortal and are aging. I am not sure what is more depressing: my gynecologist telling me that my ovaries were not "as vibrant as they once were at peak fertility" or that my biological clock was no longer. Just as everything else ages—our skin, our heart, our lungs—so, too, do our ovaries. The ovaries, in particular, are what Jennifer Garrison, a professor at the Buck Institute for Research on Aging, calls "the pacemaker of aging" for women, because they are the first organs to functionally decline with age. "Essentially, we have allowed women's health as a whole to be pigeonholed through the lens of fertility," she said in an article for *Vox*. "But the ovaries sit at the center of a complex molecular signaling network that doesn't just guide the creation of new life." Fascinating, right? But it is also disturbing, because the medical community (including myself) wasn't taught that fact years ago. This has come out only recently, which underscores how much research still needs to be done and how much we still don't know about this organ system. We have to think of our ovaries as a spoke on the menopause wheel, because they drive a lot of the symptoms we start experiencing in middle age. But that doesn't mean the wheel is broken—there is much we can do to slow ovarian aging.

Our ovaries are magical machines, although they measure barely larger than the size of an olive. To think they are ground zero for our egg production—and all human life—can be a dizzying thought. But some studies show they age two to five times faster than our other organs—and we don't know why. As life expectancy increases worldwide, ovarian aging will gradually become a major health problem for women.

We all feel that aging in different ways. Kristin, a forty-two-year-old accountant, came to see me as she was exhibiting signs of perimenopause. We went over her history, and she told me her mom went into menopause early. Her family history also included weight issues, and Kristin herself was obese (her BMI was over 30). A former smoker, she had noticed a steady weight gain over the previous two years, especially around the abdomen. It didn't help that her job was sedentary. Her perimenopausal symptoms were coming in hot, literally: She experienced hot flashes and night sweats. She also complained of irritability and anxiety, joint pain—particularly in knees and lower back—bloating, low libido, and irregular cycles. Her lifestyle may have contributed to the severity of the symptoms: Her daily food intake was predominantly ultraprocessed foods, she didn't get much exercise, she was a former smoker, and her sleep was in desperate need of an overhaul, made worse by her night sweats—a sure sign that her ovaries were aging faster than the average perimenopausal female's. Add in her family history and she had the perfect storm of ovarian aging for earlier menopause.

Ovarian aging and **senescence** are critical processes that significantly affect female reproductive health, fertility, and overall aging. Ovarian aging is the gradual decline in the number and quality of ovarian follicles (which contain eggs), while cellular senescence involves a state in which cells lose the ability to divide and function properly. These processes are interconnected and play a pivotal role in determining reproductive lifespan and overall health in women. What drives this aging process is the biological clock we discussed in the first chapter. It's really attuned to our ovaries, and it drives the aging in our bodies as females. Those beginning stages of perimenopause symptoms—less circulating progesterone, the onslaught of anxiety and depression, insomnia, the crime-scene bleeds, all of which make us miserable—are the natural process of aging at work, whether we like it or not. The more we understand that our ovaries really are driving a lot of the symptoms we start experiencing in middle age, the better we can mitigate those dreaded symptoms.

It's All About the Eggs

Women are born with a finite number of oocytes (eggs), approximately one to two million at birth. Like many good things in life, this number declines steadily over the years due to ovulation and the gradual degeneration of follicles. By the time a woman reaches puberty, around 300,000 to 500,000 oocytes remain, and by the time she enters menopause (around age fifty), only a few hundred to a thousand eggs are left.

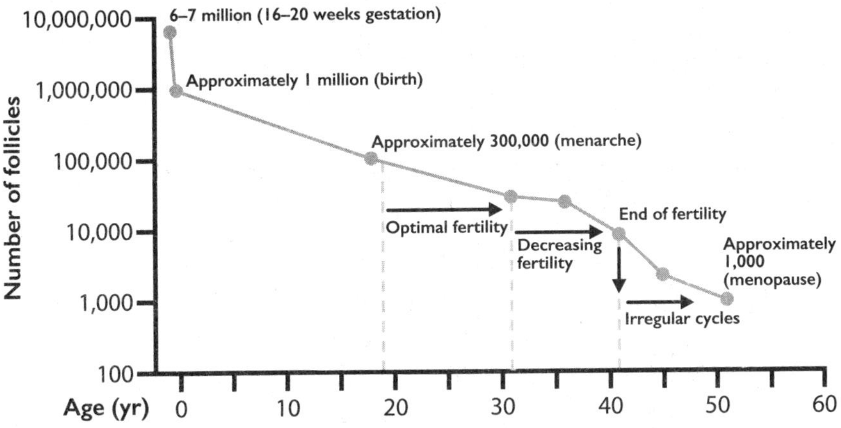

Source: https://www.medicalnewstoday.com/articles/how-many-eggs-does-a-woman-have

With aging, the quality of oocytes also declines. Aging eggs are more prone to chromosomal abnormalities, which can increase the risk of miscarriage, infertility, or congenital conditions such as Down syndrome. This is why pregnancy complications increase with age, and a parental age of thirty-five or older may be considered a higher-risk pregnancy, or the dreaded advanced maternal age (AMA). (Don't fret, I had my second pregnancy at thirty-six and found that AMA designation next to my name hilarious.)

Ovarian follicles are another marker of aging. Each of these small fluid-filled sacs contains one developing egg. Each month one egg follicle is selected (we have no idea how), and between days six and fourteen, that follicle will secrete follicle-stimulating hormone (FSH) to help the egg to mature. Around day fourteen, it releases luteinizing hormone (LH), which causes the ovary to release the egg (ovulation). With time, ovarian reserve declines in both the quantity and quality of follicles.

Imagine the ovaries are like a basket of eggs. When a girl hits puberty and starts getting her period, her body uses one egg a month. As time goes by, there are fewer eggs in the basket and some of those eggs are not as viable as they once were. When the ovaries run out of eggs, or the quality or quantity of the eggs is impacted, it can be harder for a woman to become pregnant. It can also lead to other changes in her body, such as irregular menstrual cycles, recurrent pregnancy loss, autoimmune issues, endometriosis, and ultimately menopause.

What Does Ovarian Aging (Senescence) Look Like?

What I just described, my friend, is what ovarian aging looks like. Menopause is the hallmark event of natural ovarian aging, or senescence, as we like to say in the medical field, just to make it more complicated. What does aging mean for those organs? Our ovaries house our eggs, and we are all born with a finite number of them; when they run out, we don't need to ovulate anymore, and that production shutdown ushers in menopause. Our ovaries go out of business and retire. Remember how the ovaries are like a basket of eggs that a girl is born with? Over time, the eggs get used up, and eventually, the basket is empty or the eggs become less viable.

When ovarian senescence happens, the ovaries stop releasing eggs, which causes a woman to stop having periods. No ovulation, no releasing eggs, no periods, no more babies. It's a hard fact that when we get older, typically in our early fifties, our ovaries "retire" from their job, and we go into menopause.

The Stages of Ovarian Aging and Senescence

Perimenopause and Menopause

- Ovarian senescence leads to perimenopause, during which hormonal fluctuations cause symptoms like hot flashes, night sweats, mood changes, and irregular periods.
- Eventually, menopause occurs, marked by a full year from the cessation of menstruation and the end of a woman's reproductive years. This can be made more complicated if a woman is on long-acting reversible contraceptives (LARCs) like oral contraceptives, has an IUD, or has had an ablation or hysterectomy and doesn't have monthly cycles. That's when a bit of detective work is in order to determine when this menopausal transition occurs or has occurred.
- At this time, our body continues to make a weaker form of estrogen (estrone, or E1) as estradiol stops, and our adrenals pick up the slack for progesterone (which explains why we are less stress-resilient in perimenopause—the adrenals are working in multiple capacities).

Postmenopause

- After menopause, the ovaries no longer produce significant amounts of estrogen and progesterone, leading to long-term health risks such as osteoporosis and sarcopenia, increased risk of cardiovascular disease, and changes in body composition (such as increased abdominal, or visceral, fat).
- Hormonal decline also affects skin health, cognitive function, and mood.

What Can Hasten Ovarian Aging?

There are several biological forces in our body that can hasten our ovaries' demise. Let's look at a few of these factors:

Mitochondrial aging: We are learning that the basis of ovarian aging is mitochondrial dysfunction. Mitochondria are the little powerhouses of our cells that start to work less efficiently as we age; the same applies to our ovaries. There are more mitochondria in our ovaries than in any other organ, including our brains, heart, and liver, and so when they age, so do our ovaries.

Hormonal changes: As the ovarian reserve diminishes, hormonal changes occur, including a decline in estrogen, progesterone, and, in some women, testosterone levels. This hormonal shift contributes to irregular menstrual cycles, infertility, and symptoms associated with perimenopause and menopause.

Genetics: Our ancestry can play a big part in how and when we start menopause. Black women tend to start menopause about six to eight months earlier than white women, and their symptoms can be longer-lasting and more intense. Hispanic women have also been shown to have earlier onset of menopause, while Asian women tend to go through menopause a little bit later. In 1994, the pivotal Study of Women's Health Across the Nation (SWAN) was published, and their findings—after following 3,300 women for decades—confirmed that Black women experience symptoms for ten or more years, nearly double the time white and Asian women experience them.

What Lifestyle Choices Accelerate This Process for Women?

Our ovaries all have a predetermined shelf life, but our lifestyle choices can play a part in shortening or extending that lifespan.

We know that approximately 5 percent of women will enter menopause early, between the ages of forty and forty-five. Menopause occurring before the age of forty is described as premature and occurs in approximately 1 percent of women. Here, you'll see many of the usual suspects that may hasten our ovaries' demise.

Poor nutrition: We know eating a less processed, more nutrient-dense diet supports a healthy body, while an ultraprocessed, nutrient-deficient diet can accelerate aging. This also applies to our ovaries, which are especially important as the pacemakers of our bodies. The science shows that our ovarian reserve appears to be influenced by what we eat. A high BMI has a negative impact on our ovaries, decreasing follicle count and anti-Mullerian hormone (AMH) levels. (The AMH hormone is produced in our ovarian follicles and can reflect a decline in ovarian function and efficacy.) According to the authors of the Moli-sani Study, ultraprocessed foods have non-nutrient ingredients that may harm human health beyond their low nutritional content. The researchers found that a diet with more than 14 percent of total calories from ultraprocessed foods was linked to accelerated biological aging, and that the toxic by-products and endocrine-mimicking chemicals in the packaging of these foods caused further hormone dysregulation. Materials like bisphenol A and phthalates can be absorbed by the ultraprocessed foods, especially when they're stored for long periods. These chemicals are known to induce and promote hormone dysregulation and oxidative stress, which over time can lead to insulin resistance and promote inflammation—the basis of nearly all chronic diseases.

Stress: Too much stress can affect the body, including the ovaries, in many ways. Managing stress by relaxing, having fun, and sleeping well can help the ovaries stay healthy. Recall that long-term high cortisol can age our bodies. When I talked to Kristin, I found out that she had grown up in the inner city with a great deal of childhood stressors, including an absent father. Several studies have indicated an association between disadvantaged childhood socioeconomic position and earlier menopause. One of the most crucial factors defining the quality of childhood environment is the experience of adversities such as psychological stress or trauma, poverty, abuse, or neglect. Kristin had all of the above. (We'll get more into ACEs and their devastating effects on our health in chapter 9.)

Smoking: We know that smoking is bad for the whole body, including the ovaries, but it is also the strongest and most clearly demonstrated risk factor for early menopause. Kristin had started smoking cigarettes as a teen and only quit a few years prior, and she mentioned that her mom had smoked during her pregnancy and had exposed Kristin to secondhand smoke during her childhood. It has been hypothesized that prenatal exposure to cigarette smoke may affect the follicle pool by altering the development of ovarian follicles (this is intergenerational, meaning it is inheritable); the median age at menopause was 1.2 years younger for current smokers compared with nonsmokers.

Alcohol: Sorry, ladies, drinking excessively can accelerate aging everywhere, and that means in the ovaries as well. We may tolerate alcohol in our twenties and thirties, but I find that most, if not all, women need to change their relationship with it in perimenopause and menopause. While mechanisms driving the relationship between alcohol intake and menopause are not fully understood, studies show that higher consumption of alcohol is related to experiencing menopause at a younger age. This could be caused by inflammation and oxidative stress that induces higher levels of FSH, which may be associated with ovarian damage or acceleration of aging. Long-term moderate alcohol consumption also may lead to diminished ovarian reserve.

Lack of exercise: Staying active and exercising regularly can help the ovaries stay healthy longer. Being sedentary or not moving enough could lead to problems in the body, including, yep, you guessed it, the ovaries. One study demonstrated that moderate physical activity is associated with improved age-specific levels of ovarian reserve markers, including FSH, AMH, and antral follicle count (AFC) levels. Exercise of course improves insulin sensitivity, helps maintain muscle mass (specifically strength training), and contributes to improved sleep quality and overall health, so this will help slow ovarian aging as well. (We'll talk about the importance of exercise in chapter 7 of this book.)

Endocrine disruptors: Endocrine-disrupting chemicals (EDCs)—chemicals that can interfere with our body's hormone system—can be found nearly everywhere. From BPA in our water bottles to phthalates in our makeup to polyfluoroalkyl substances (PFAS) in our nonstick cookware and stain-resistant furniture, all of these disrupt our body's general reproductive health and, in particular, accelerate ovarian aging. EDCs can also impair follicular development and even disrupt the creation of our hormones during ovarian aging. (We'll cover these a bit more in chapter 6.)

Excess weight: Obesity and excess body fat can lead to insulin resistance and metabolic issues that will affect us, especially how we age and how our ovaries age. Recently, studies have shown an association between adipose tissue, or body fat, and ovarian aging. Being obese (with a BMI over 30) can contribute to early ovarian aging, and egg quality can be reduced. Excess body fat can accelerate follicle development and loss and potentially lead to premature ovarian insufficiency, or POI. There has been a connection between obesity, oocyte changes, and the gut microbiome as well; sometimes this manifests as polycystic ovarian syndrome (PCOS), which we talk about later in this chapter.

Post-cancers and 'ectomies: A partial hysterectomy can hasten menopause and ovarian aging by four years.

The earlier you transition into menopause, the longer your body is forced to live without the benefit of your natural estrogen, progesterone, and, in some instances, testosterone, and the less healthy you're going to be. Mental health, cardiovascular disease, insulin resistance, and obesity risks all go up. Women who are experiencing an earlier menopause should see their health provider and find out what appropriate treatment they can start to allay such health risk.

All that said, it is not all doom and gloom! And there are simple and proactive ways we can mitigate these risks. With Kristin, I had her stop smoking (slowly), started her on key supplements like urolithin A, and had her do three days of sixteen-hour intermittent fasting each week, all in an effort to improve her microbiome. In terms of exercise, she was very reluctant to make changes all at once, so we just took baby steps. She started walking after meals, about ten to fifteen minutes, then she added in two or three days a week of a body-weight strength training (think squats and lunges). After a few months, she definitely saw an improvement in her body and saw the scale moving in the right direction. She had more energy. She was starting to sleep better. Some of the brain fog that she was experiencing lifted.

Like Clockwork

You read earlier that you have inner clocks—tiny timers throughout the body that help control when things happen, such as when you feel sleepy, hungry, or full of energy. Your ovaries have them, too, keeping time on how hormones like estrogen fluctuate on a daily, weekly, and monthly basis. These hormone cycles in turn affect the gut microbiome, and together they regulate hormones, digestion, and energy levels, which are important for health and overall well-being.

For example, changes in estrogen can influence the balance of bacteria in the gut, and our ovarian clock genes help keep this balance on track. But if the body's clocks get out of sync—say, from staying up too late, eating at odd times, or experiencing stress—it can affect not only our master clock but also the clocks throughout our entire body, including our gut bacteria and microbiome. This might lead to a myriad of health issues, including digestive problems or hormone imbalances. In females, this can also impact the menstrual cycle and how the ovaries function and age.

The Gut–Ovary Axis

There's more to the connection between the gut and the ovaries than the clocks going haywire. Recent studies have suggested a connection between ovarian aging and the gut microbiota, and their interaction is bidirectional, meaning there's a clear communication superhighway between our ovaries and our gut microbiome. So, the makeup and diversity of our gut microbiota have profound consequences on ovarian function. And because it is believed that our ovaries set the pace for our overall aging, well, that means they can set the pace for our gut microbiota as well.

Here's how it works:

1. **Gut bacteria and hormones:** The bacteria in your gut help manage hormones like estrogen. Estrogen is crucial for your ovarian function, so the healthier your gut bacteria are, the better they can help keep your hormone levels balanced.
2. **Ovaries and the gut:** In return, the ovaries produce hormones that affect not just the ovaries themselves but also the bacteria in your gut. These hormones can help certain types of bacteria grow, keeping the gut microbiome healthy.

The beauty of symbiosis! It's the ol' "I'll scratch your back and you scratch mine" motto. The gut bacteria help the ovaries by managing hormones, and the ovaries help the gut by supporting its bacteria. Together, they keep important things in your body running smoothly, like your hormones and your overall health!

Dr. Lisa Mosconi, a leading neuroscientist and women's brain-health specialist, talks about the three key times in a woman's life when our bodies change dramatically: puberty, pregnancy, and perimenopause. It shouldn't be a surprise to you by now that the gut microbiome is no different. During puberty, a lot of changes happen in a young woman's body, including in the gut microbiome. When puberty starts, hormones like estrogen begin to increase, and these hormones can affect the balance of bacteria in the gut.

The gut microbiome sees a lot of action during puberty. First, estrogen and other hormones increase, which can cause shifts in the types and amounts of bacteria in the gut. Some bacteria respond to these hormone changes and might grow more, while others decrease. The types of bacteria in the gut can become more varied during puberty. This is usually a good thing because having a more diverse microbiome helps keep the gut and body healthy—and better arms our immune system, helping the body more effectively fight off illnesses and stay healthy. We see an impact on metabolism, too, as changes in gut bacteria might also affect how the body breaks down food and absorbs nutrients, which can play a role in weight and energy levels. In short, puberty brings changes to the gut microbiome, with hormones like estrogen causing shifts in the types of bacteria that live in the gut. These changes help support the body's growth and health during this important time.

As we have learned, during menopause, there are changes to the microbiome's composition (again) and microbial diversity. These changes are so significant that they start to resemble what a male's microbiome looks like before puberty. Amazing, right? However, these changes are not always to our benefit, as less circulating estrogen, in particular, sets the stage for inflammation, oxidative stress, and increased susceptibility to dysbiosis (the "weeds in the garden" analogy), ultimately making us more likely to develop a leaky gut.

POI

Premature ovarian insufficiency (POI), formerly called premature ovarian failure (POF), is a condition in which a woman's ovaries stop working properly before age forty. POI develops in about 1 percent of women. It has serious health consequences, and women who lose ovarian function at a young age are at an increased risk for cognitive dysfunction, autoimmune and thyroid disease, cardiovascular disease, osteopenia, osteoporosis, infertility, genitourinary syndrome of menopause, and premature death.

Mounting evidence suggests that GM dysbiosis (the lack of good bacteria) is associated with POI. For reasons not yet fully understood, the ovaries don't make enough estrogen or release eggs regularly, which can lead to infertility. Causes of POI include genetics (Turner syndrome), significant eating disorders, autoimmune disorders like Hashimoto's thyroiditis, and even vaccines, with some research suggesting an association with the HPV vaccine.

POI can sometimes be confused with premature menopause, but they aren't the same. Women with POI can still have periods (they may be irregular) and can get pregnant (although it is very rare). With premature menopause, women are done with their periods, can no longer get pregnant, and have follicle depletion, and they tend to be younger than forty-five years old.

What's Ovarian Aging Got to Do with Leaky Gut?

Leaky gut. It doesn't paint a pretty image, does it? Remember that in a healthy gut, the lining acts as a barrier, allowing necessary nutrients to be absorbed into the bloodstream while keeping out harmful substances like toxins, undigested food particles, and bacteria. If the gut weakens from chronic exposure to foods and medications that irritate it, gaps can form in these tight junctions, and you can develop a leaky gut. When this happens, fragments of protein and bacteria that aren't supposed to can get into your system and create all sorts of trouble. It is important to note that leaky gut is typically caused by a cumulative effect. One indulgence in processed foods or a short dose of antibiotics is not typically the issue; it is the long-term choices that we make. If you have leaky gut, you may experience one or many of these symptoms:

- Digestive issues, such as gas, bloating, diarrhea, or constipation
- Food sensitivities
- Irregular menstrual cycles
- Fatigue
- Low libido
- Joint pain and muscle aches
- Skin issues, such as acne, eczema, or psoriasis
- Autoimmune conditions, such as Hashimoto's thyroiditis, rheumatoid arthritis, or lupus
- Trouble sleeping
- Anxiety, depression, or moodiness
- Bacterial overgrowth, such as candida overgrowth or SIBO (small intestinal bacterial overgrowth)
- Weight-loss resistance

Leaky gut can become more prevalent during menopause because of hormonal changes, particularly the decline in estrogen, which plays a role in maintaining the integrity of the gut lining. This estrogen loss can weaken tight junctions between our gut cells, or enterocytes, allowing toxins and pathogens to pass through into the bloodstream. This can lead to systemic inflammation, cause food sensitivities, and contribute to perimenopausal symptoms such as fatigue, mood swings, and metabolic issues. Additionally, gut microbiome changes during menopause can further exacerbate leaky gut.

Now that you know about leaky gut, we are going to elevate things and talk about microbial translocation. This is just a fancy phrase for what happens when leaky gut not only lets toxins and pathogens through its lining but also allows microbes to translocate (a.k.a. move) from the gut to systemic circulation. This activates our immune system and its sister, inflammation. Both estrogen and progesterone help maintain the gut barrier and are master regulators of the immune system. So, with the onset of menopause, we see a reduction in barrier integrity and increasing microbial translocation in the gut, though few studies have examined the association of menopause with gut barrier integrity and microbial translocation in humans.

PCOS

Yes, here's another acronym. But this may be one you have heard of before: Polycystic ovarian syndrome (PCOS) is the most common endocrine disorder in women of reproductive age, but it affects women's health and quality of life across their lives. Depending on which study you believe, PCOS affects roughly 8 to 13 percent of us.

The cause is not fully understood, but it is commonly thought to be a combination of hormonal imbalances and metabolic factors. Women with PCOS often have higher levels of androgens (male hormones), such as testosterone, which can disrupt ovulation (leading to irregular or missed

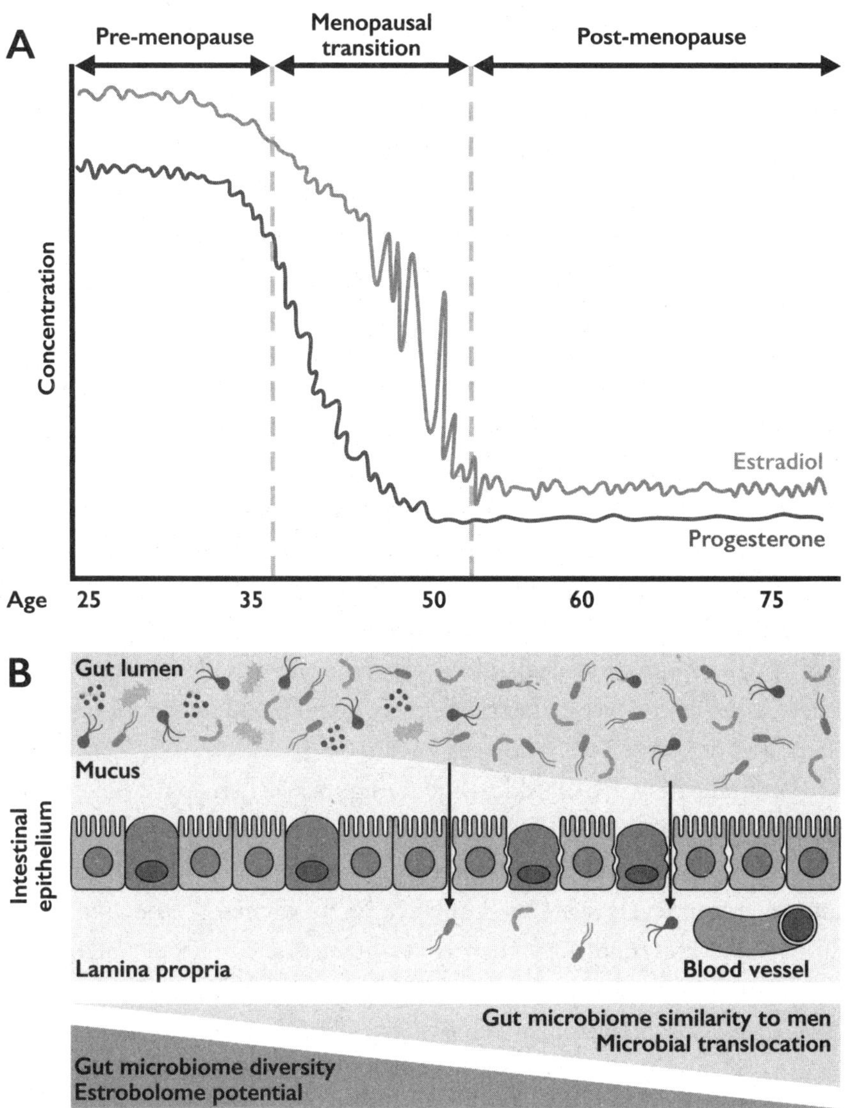

Microbial translocation activates the immune system, causing inflammation, and is implicated in the development of many diseases, including IBD and HIV.

Source: https://pmc.ncbi.nlm.nih.gov/articles/PMC9379122/figure/f0002/

periods or extreme and very heavy periods), cause excessive body hair growth (but also scalp hair thinning) or acne, and contribute to infertility issues. While it can cause weight gain (especially around the waist), nearly a quarter of women with PCOS are not overweight.

Diane was one of those women. She had been diagnosed with PCOS when she and her husband had been trying to conceive many years before. She was part of the 25 percent of women who are thin with PCOS (what we call a thin-phenotype). Most women with PCOS are characteristically overweight or obese. She assumed that her issues would "work themselves out" prior to menopause, but they didn't. Her perimenopause journey was marked by worsening anxiety, depression, insomnia, and wild fluctuations in estrogen, along with weight gain, breast tenderness, and heavy menstrual cycles. She felt awful. She developed insulin resistance and high blood pressure, and she became more sensitive to what she ate, especially processed foods. I helped her map out a plan to lower her blood sugar, suggesting GLP-1, as well as encouraging a low-carb diet, strength training, and walking after meals. Oral progesterone was also added. Guess what. After several weeks, her sleep, energy, and mood improved substantially, and her weight went down.

Unfortunately, PCOS doesn't just disappear when you're navigating perimenopause into menopause. In fact, androgen levels are known to remain stable or even increase as women enter menopause, while at the same time, estrogen levels decrease dramatically. As women become more androgenic, several conditions, such as insulin resistance, chronic inflammation, increasing abdominal fat, and lipid abnormalities, tend to worsen. Although ovarian androgen secretion capacity declines with age in both healthy women and women with PCOS, it remains enhanced in most PCOS patients until the late reproductive years.

Unfortunately, when a woman goes through menopause, it does not mean that her PCOS goes away; quite the contrary. Just like Diane, women with a history of PCOS are at a greater risk of unfavorable hormonal and metabolic changes related to menopause, which means they're also exposed to greater health risks. Additionally, patients with PCOS have higher rates of adverse reproductive, cardiovascular, psychological, metabolic, and neoplastic outcomes than the general female population.

PCOS and the Gut Microbiome

The gut microbiome in patients with PCOS often shows unique differences compared to those without the condition. These can play a role in the development and severity of PCOS symptoms. Here's what makes the gut microbiome in PCOS patients unique:

- **Reduced diversity of gut bacteria:** PCOS patients tend to have fewer types of beneficial bacteria in their gut. A diverse microbiome is important for overall health, and lower diversity can lead to imbalances that may worsen inflammation and hormone imbalances.
- **Increased "bad" bacteria:** Studies have found that PCOS patients often have higher levels of harmful or inflammatory bacteria. These bacteria can produce toxins that contribute to low-grade inflammation, which can worsen PCOS symptoms like insulin resistance and weight gain.
- **Dysbiosis:** PCOS is often linked to dysbiosis, which means an imbalance between good and bad bacteria. This imbalance can affect how the body processes hormones like estrogen and androgens (which are often elevated in PCOS).
- **Dysregulation in the gut–brain axis:** This can lead to dysregulation of gastrointestinal hormones, including GLP-1, which can delay gastric emptying, impacting satiety signaling and weight goals. In PCOS, GLP-1 levels tend to be lower than normal.
- **Leaky gut:** PCOS patients are more likely to experience leaky gut, which can increase inflammation and worsen PCOS symptoms.
- **Increased insulin resistance:** The gut microbiome plays a role in how the body processes sugars and regulates insulin. Fifty to 70 percent of PCOS patients have insulin resistance to varying degrees, especially those with obesity. In PCOS, gut bacteria imbalances may contribute to insulin resistance, a key factor in the condition.

- **Altered production of SCFAs:** As we learned in chapter 1, SCFAs, produced by gut bacteria, are essential for gut health and metabolism. PCOS patients often have lower levels of SCFAs, which can contribute to weight gain and poor metabolic health.
- **Hormonal imbalances:** The gut microbiome helps regulate estrogen levels by breaking it down and recycling it. In PCOS, gut imbalances can lead to higher androgen levels and lower estrogen, contributing to symptoms like irregular periods and excess hair growth.

So, with this information, you can appreciate why having PCOS is significant even before the transition into menopause, and its impact on the microbiome.

Specific Challenges in Menopausal Females with PCOS

As it happens, the lipid abnormalities worsen as women with PCOS age, especially with regard to triglyceride and high-density lipoprotein (HDL) concentrations. Long-term exposure to elevated androgen levels in women with PCOS can cause excessive facial and body hair, hair loss, and even balding that extends past menopause, not to mention weight-loss resistance. Inflammation and metabolic health markers also worsen with age in women with PCOS (as hs-CRP and glucose/insulin labs would show), which can lead to systemic metabolic disorders, such as hyperinsulinemia and insulin resistance (IR). PCOS patients also have to worry about obesity, increased risk of type 2 diabetes, and cardiovascular disease. It's not surprising these issues may impact self-esteem throughout a woman's life, but while she needs to be extra diligent in following a healthy lifestyle and, in particular, maintaining a healthy body weight as she enters menopause, there is a promising way forward, and we will discuss this further in part 2.

Now that we've talked about the ovaries, the driver of female aging, let's look into the effects they have on our hormones, and of course, how it all relates back to our gut.

Chapter Summary

1. Our ovaries are the pacemakers of aging for our entire body.
2. We are born with a finite number of eggs that decreases sharply after age thirty.
3. Lifestyle choices can positively or negatively impact when we transition into menopause.
4. The gut–ovary axis is these two systems constantly interacting with one another to optimize our health.

References for this chapter can be found on my website: cynthiathurlow.com/themenopausegut-references

Chapter 4

Don't Tell Me I'm Hormonal

Danielle, a forty-five-year-old mom of three kids, came to me because her periods were becoming close to, as she put it, a "crime scene":

> I finally was in a good place with navigating middle age, and then *boom*. I started getting frequent, heavy cycles. . . . I bled through my pants. I felt like I was back in middle school and hadn't yet learned the art of that time of the month. I would have to double up on a tampon *and* a pad just to be safe.

Heavy bleeding wasn't the only problem she was battling. She also had tender breasts for most of her cycle, and she had no libido—no energy for anything, really. She was transitioning into perimenopause, when our ovaries begin to produce less progesterone and start to peter out, much like that car engine that's on its last legs. When that happens, significant hormone fluctuations begin, wreaking havoc on our once-stable system.

This doesn't always show up as heavy cycles—actually, the opposite can happen, too, in the later stages of perimenopause. Cassandra, age fifty, noticed her periods were becoming less regular and much lighter. She was having increasing bouts of constipation, gas, and bloating. She tried to eat healthy, but that was hard to do when she usually ate while driving or doing errands. She noticed the telltale sign of her pants feeling tight; her scale seemed to be going in the wrong direction. Cassandra and Danielle were each feeling the effects of their own personal roller-coaster ride of hormone levels during perimenopause, creating symptoms such as weight gain, loss of libido, painful sex, and crazy moods.

We have talked about hormones—those critical chemical messengers that play a role in regulating nearly every function of our body—throughout this book, but in this chapter, we'll really get into how they work and interact with our immune system, gut, and brain, and what happens when they decrease as we age. Our sex hormones—specifically estrogen, progesterone, and, to a lesser extent, testosterone—make us who we are as women. (Note: We have a tenth of the testosterone of men, but it is super potent.) These tiny messengers tell different parts of our body what to do, like grow, create a baby, get more energy, or feel emotion. Cortisol and insulin factor into our health, too. For most of our lives, they strike a balance within our body; when change happens, though—ahem, that middle-age transition—our hormone levels also change, and we see seismic shifts in our physical makeup.

Let's unpack these tiny wonders and see how they work in tandem with our gut, and we can better mitigate their inevitable retreat.

Estrogen Basics

In the symphony of sex hormones, our estrogens are queen. Produced by our ovaries from our first period until menopause, they have more than four hundred crucial roles in the most important parts of our bodies, such as our heart, brain, bone, muscles, bladder, gut, uterus, ovaries, vagina, and brain. They aid in regulating insulin sensitivity; maintaining bone density, skin health, collagen production, and a healthy gut microbiome; and controlling inflammation. But did you know that while we think of estrogen as one hormone, there are actually three main types in the body?

Estrone (E1) is the primary estrogen found in the body *after* menopause. It's a weaker form of estrogen compared with estradiol (E2), and it can be converted to estradiol when needed. Estrone is produced in smaller amounts by adipose (fat) tissue and the adrenal glands, especially after the ovaries stop producing estradiol at menopause. Dr. Pam Smith, the founder of the Fellowship in Anti-Aging, Regenerative, and Functional Medicine, believes that estrone produced in fat tissue may have a role in modulating the loss of bone mass after menopause. Quick fact: The more body fat you have, the more E1 your body makes. Because it is produced in fat tissue, this hormone is responsible for some of the body composition changes we experience in perimenopause and beyond, such as getting "fluffy" around the middle. Until menopause, we primarily house subcutaneous fat (fat that is just below the skin) around our butt, thighs, and hips, but this shifts at this stage of life. After menopause we tend to accumulate a different type of fat, called visceral fat, which sits deeper in our abdomen. Because of its vicinity to important organs, this fat can make us more prone to inflammation, insulin resistance, heart disease, and some cancers.

Estradiol (E2) is the most common type of estrogen in women of reproductive age, starting when we get our first period and slowing down when those periods finally stop. Produced in the ovaries, it plays a crucial role in regulating the menstrual cycle, supporting reproductive health, maintaining bone density, and controlling the growth of the endometrial lining from menarche to menopause. Its levels fluctuate throughout the menstrual cycle and are highest during the reproductive years. In perimenopause, wildly fluctuating levels of estradiol can show up as heavier menstrual cycles, weight-loss resistance, brain fog, shorter cycles, insomnia, night sweats, PMS, and headaches. Low E2 also makes it harder to fight off infections—this helps explain why we are so susceptible to infections in perimenopause and menopause.

Estriol (E3) is the weakest of the three types and is primarily produced during pregnancy. It is made by the placenta and helps support the growth and development of the fetus. Estriol levels are evident in all women but typically very low in nonpregnant women.

Key Benefits of Estrogen

1. Regulates appetite
2. Maintains health of gut microbiome
3. Maintains immune system and modulates inflammation
4. Increases lean body mass
5. Reduces abdominal fat
6. Improves insulin sensitivity
7. Reduces blood pressure
8. Maintains bone density
9. Improves mood/sleep
10. Maintains cognition

Signs of High Estrogen

1. Weight gain
2. Heavy cycles
3. Breast tenderness
4. Headaches
5. Changes in libido
6. Bloating, fatigue, insomnia
7. Irritability, mood swings
8. Insomnia

Signs of Low Estrogen

1. Brain fog
2. Itchy ears
3. Dry skin
4. Weight issues
5. Joint pain
6. GSM

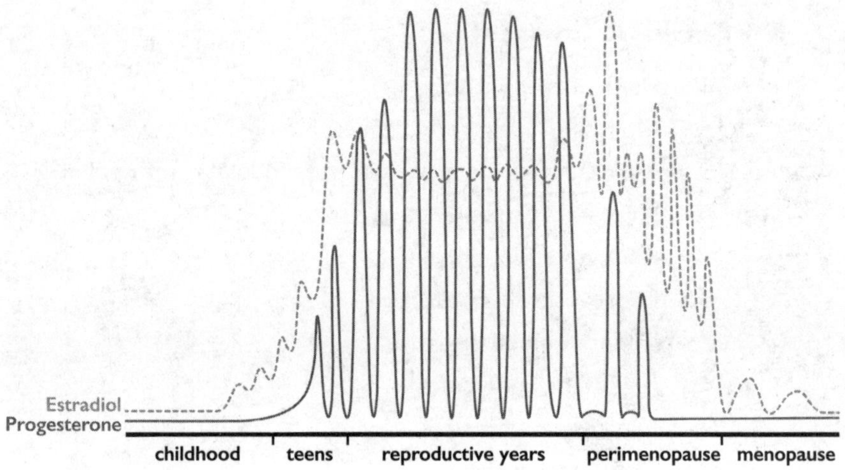

Source: https://wellfemme.com.au/understanding-hormonal-changes-during-menopause/

Greek to Me

Hold on, we aren't quite done yet. Estrogen has two key receptors to bind to receptor sites in our body: estrogen receptor alpha and estrogen receptor beta. Sounds Greek to you, right? Well, it is, but to help you understand them a bit better, I like to use a car analogy: Alpha promotes cell growth and regulates genes and cell membranes, while beta slows cell growth, so think of alpha as the car's gas pedal and beta as the brakes. Speed up or slow down, that's their job. They work together to keep our body in homeostasis.

Like estrogen, these receptors are present throughout our bodies, but in different concentrations—in our brain, the lining of our intestines, lungs, kidneys, heart, hair follicles, bones, adrenal glands, skin . . . pretty much everywhere. Alpha also intersects with the innate immune system, while beta works closely with the hormone oxytocin (found in the brain/gut/vagus nerve) and plays an important role in digestion and supporting the parasympathetic part of our autonomic nervous system. And guess what. Lower estrogen means that these receptors work less efficiently. During perimenopause, when estrogen levels fluctuate and the balance of estrogen and progesterone becomes dysregulated, it can show up as heavy menses, sore breasts, weight-loss resistance, poor sleep, moodiness, and more.

How Does Estrogen Impact the Immune System?

We talked earlier about how estrogen influences the number, activity, and function of all immune cells in both innate and adaptive immune responses. The menopausal loss of estrogen as an immune modulator means that our chances of chronic inflammation increase as we age. Simply put, with this loss of estrogen, our bodily functions aren't as well balanced and don't work as efficiently. Again, think of an older car. It still drives, but its engine may go, and you may need new brake pads or a paint job; generally, we have to be more conscientious about maintenance. The same thing applies to our body as it ages and estrogen declines. We have to be more conscientious about regular checkups and lifestyle choices.

The takeaway: The loss of estrogen in the late stages of perimenopause and menopause has a profound impact on how our bodies react to opportunistic infections and leads to more inflammation and more cytokines. (Remember, those cytokine storms make it hard for the body to heal because the immune system is causing more damage.)

GENITOURINARY SYNDROME OF MENOPAUSE, OR GSM

This sexy name is for all those symptoms we feel "down there" in midlife: (a) genital symptoms like dryness, irritation, burning, itching, and abnormal vaginal discharge; (b) sexual symptoms like lack of lubrication, discomfort, and dyspareunia (pain during intercourse); and (c) urinary symptoms like urgency, increased frequency, discomfort while urinating, incontinence, and recurrent urinary tract infections. Approximately 40 to 50 percent of women in menopause and 15 percent of perimenopausal women are affected. Changes are due to the loss of estrogen and its impact on the delicate vaginal microbiome, which in turn impacts the pH; and the loss of lactobacilli, which help with mucus production and lubrication. Vaginal estrogen can address these symptoms, along with DHEA or testosterone supplements.

How Does Estrogen Impact Circadian Clocks?

Recall that circadian clocks govern our entire lives on a twenty-four-hour schedule, and our main master clock is the SCN (suprachiasmatic nucleus), which is controlled by many factors, including sex hormones, like estrogen. So it is reasonable to conclude that when estrogen levels go down, it will disrupt the natural order of our inner clock. An animal model study demonstrated that low estrogen can drive disruption in the circadian rhythm. Disruption in circadian clocks and lowered estrogen levels mean poor sleep, putting women in middle age at risk for developing insulin resistance, diabetes, and obesity.

We also talked about misalignment in our circadian rhythm when we get poor sleep and what that means to our health, but it bears repeating here. The risks are well studied—so much so that in 2007, the International Agency for Research on Cancer (IARC) classified shift work as a probable human carcinogen. All those hardworking ER nurses and doctors, caregivers, police officers, EMS workers, bus drivers, and others who work night shifts and disrupt their inner clocks have a greater risk of inflammation and disease.

Finding the Right Balance

You now know that we have estrogen receptors *everywhere*, including our GI tract, which encompasses the lining of our intestines. When we have enough estrogen, our gut microbiota displays species diversity, because there is a bidirectional relationship between estrogen and the microbiome. If our estrogen levels are healthy and well maintained, we have better beneficial bacteria levels and improved microbial diversity. During perimenopause and menopause, fluctuations in estrogen negatively impact both beneficial bacteria levels *and* microbial diversity, and we are at greater risk for a leaky gut. Developing a leaky gut can make us more susceptible to inflammation, dysbiosis, activation of T cells, and creation of food sensitivities (food particles leak into our bloodstream, creating an immune response); as a result, we will experience bloating, nausea, brain fog, joint pain, gas, and dyspepsia, as well as constipation. Not fun.

However, there is also such a thing as too much estrogen. Hormones are regulated predominantly by the liver and then our intestines, which typically package up the estrogen that we don't need so we can poop it out. If things are not working properly, we will recirculate the estrogen that our bodies should have eliminated in our poop, which can exacerbate symptoms of high estrogen levels.

So, here's where the estrobolome—a special group of bacteria in the gut that regulates the body's circulating estrogen—comes into play. When your body is done breaking down estrogen in the liver, it sends it to the gut to transport it out of our bodies (ideally). An enzyme found in the estrobolome called beta-glucuronidase helps control how much estrogen stays or goes. When this process is not working well, it can lead to dysbiosis and may, sadly, force us to recirculate our estrogen. Recirculating estrogen is a complicated process, but the point is that we don't want "used" estrogen in our system because it disturbs that important balance between estrogen and progesterone, which can create what we refer to as estrogen dominance. If we recirculate our estrogen, this puts us at risk for feeling pretty crummy and may lead to poor metabolic health, obesity, endometrial hyperplasia, endometriosis, and even cognitive dysfunction.

Keeping the right balance is important to help your body work properly. When our estobolome is working, our bodies are able to process estrogen and its metabolites efficiently. But many people don't properly break down estrogens (this can be caused by genetics, as in my case) and instead recirculate it, which can lead to estrogen dominance. Certain genetic mutations (like in the MTHFR [methylenetetrahydrofolate reductase] gene, which affects how the body processes folate) can impact estrogen detoxification pathways. (Don't worry if you have this; this just means being conscientious about lifestyle choices and appropriate supplementation.) Those with estrogen dominance have to work harder to help the body break down estrogen, and that includes adopting a healthy diet and lifestyle to ensure balanced beta-glucuronidase to aid in that breakdown. If people don't have properly broken-down estrogens, it can predispose them to certain diseases over time, including some types of cancers, poor metabolic health, obesity, endometriosis, polycystic ovarian syndrome, infertility, cardiovascular disease, and poor cognitive function.

Remember, we want the right amount of estrogen—not too much, not too little, like the Goldilocks effect—to optimize our health. As this starts to shift in perimenopause and menopause, we'll have to compensate for those alterations in sex hormones with good lifestyle choices.

How Does Estrogen Impact Our Brain?

If all that disruption is not enough, estrogen can mess with our brain, too. Healthy estrogen levels help reduce inflammation and also protect nerve cells that help with neuroplasticity in the brain. If there's less circulating estrogen, all these processes can be negatively impacted and can show up as brain fog, changes in executive functioning, and inability to learn as efficiently as we did when we were younger.

The hippocampus is responsible for memory consolidation, learning, and making new memories. As we navigate perimenopause into menopause, we may find it more challenging to navigate directions, remember new facts, and form new memories as our levels of estrogen fluctuate. How do these changes affect our memory? The brain has a lot of estrogen receptors, specifically for estradiol, the primary estrogen produced by the ovaries. These receptors are related to memory, cognition, and temperature regulation. This onset of cognitive problems can have a significant impact on a substantial proportion of women. Research has shown that verbal learning and memory are particularly affected during perimenopause, and new research suggests that perimenopause may also be associated with deficits in processing speed, attention, and working memory. So forgetting where you put your car keys, phone, or sunglasses is not cause for concern. Amazingly, the brain adapts to the new hormonal landscape when estrogen levels decline in perimenopause into menopause, as it can adjust the amount of estrogen receptors and make the existing receptors more sensitive to estrogen. Still, it's common to experience brain fog and other brain-related symptoms during this time.

Key to maintaining our mental cognition is trying to maintain our estrogen levels for as long as we can; research shows that if someone goes into menopause before forty, considered to be premature menopause, or goes into menopause early, typically between the ages of forty and forty-five, she is at greater risk of dementia than a woman who goes into menopause in her fifties.

Neuroscience researcher Dr. Lisa Mosconi has done incredible work in these areas. Her findings suggest that the decline in estrogen during menopause significantly affects brain regions involved in memory and cognition, potentially increasing the risk for neurodegenerative diseases like Alzheimer's (AD). This research underscores the importance of hormonal health in maintaining cognitive function as we age. Additionally, research suggests that the risk for Alzheimer's and cognitive decline is tied to our gut microbiome. We know that the risk for AD increases during the menopause transition, and that menopausal females make up 60 percent of all AD patients. One study indicates that the neuroprotective effects of estrogen help to modulate female cognitive aging. Additionally, the gut microbiota, through its breakdown of estrogens in bile, plays a role in determining systemic estrogen levels in the body; therefore, we can speculate that the gut microbiome may mediate or contribute to the decline of estrogen levels in menopausal females.

The Role Estrogen Plays in Weight Gain in Menopause

Unwanted weight gain is probably one of the most dreaded effects of perimenopause and menopause. Muffin top, bat wings, back fat—we all have those places we want to improve once we hit forty. Why is that? During this transitional time in our lives, our bodies start losing muscle mass, and this is replaced with increased fat mass. We also have more sensitivities to sleep disruption, stress, inflammatory foods, food frequency, and physical inactivity. Add in the body composition changes of muscle loss and fat gain, and shifts in hormones like estrogen and testosterone, and it is the perfect storm for weight gain and weight-loss resistance, which translates into that extra ten to fifteen pounds we can never seem to shake off.

The numbers back this up: Obesity affects 65 percent of women in menopause (yikes)! The relationship between the gut microbiota and estrogen is speculated to contribute to weight gain. Even more so, the gut microbiome is related to obesity, and menopause is associated with a higher risk of obesity.

How do we lose muscle? The gut microbiome in menopause impacts skeletal muscle mass through the synthesis of butyrate in healthy menopausal women. SCFAs activate signaling pathways (like 5'-AMP-activated protein kinase [AMPK] and mammalian target of rapamycin [mTOR]) to promote muscle protein synthesis. And certain types of SCFAs, including butyrate, have potent anti-inflammatory benefits, so fewer SCFAs means more inflammation or inflammaging and worsened insulin resistance, as well as a negative net impact on our mitochondria.

Sarcopenia, or loss of muscle mass, is a huge issue, and it's accelerated in menopause. It is thought that we lose 0.5 percent of our lean body mass (LBM) during menopause, while fat mass increases by 1.7 percent per year. Overall, we also lose 3 to 8 percent of our muscle mass each decade, and this accelerates after age sixty. (This is why it's so important to eat right—healthier microbiomes in menopausal females may make it easier to maintain and build skeletal muscle mass.)

Progesterone

Progesterone—princess to the estrogen queen—is manufactured in several places throughout the body: our ovaries, adrenal glands, brain, spinal cord, and peripheral nerves. There is significantly less research on progesterone, but we do know it primarily keeps a check on estrogen's growth and possibly increases the healthy progesterone-to-estrogen ratio we all desire.

- **Impact on sleep:** We know that the menstrual cycle is governed by the circadian clock, so it would not be too far of a stretch to assume that the shifts in progesterone and estrogen in perimenopause and menopause would impact sleep.
- **Microbial support:** Progesterone enhances gastric emptying. Again, research speaks to the bidirectional relationship between sex hormones and the gut.
- **Brain effects:** Cognitively, estrogen used with progesterone appears to protect our brains and may reverse age-dependent changes in our brains and nerves brought on by menopause. On a more emotional level, progesterone calms us down. One of its metabolites made in the brain, allopregnanolone, is a natural sedative; it delivers information to a receptor that helps increase the sensitivity of a very important neurotransmitter (GABA, or gamma-aminobutyric acid) that helps reduce anxiety. In addition, oxytocin and progesterone work synergistically to help reduce stress and promote emotional well-being. Progesterone also increases serotonin, one of our "feel-good" hormones, and reduces age-dependent changes in the brain. The perimenopause-to-menopause transition puts us at greater risk for mood disorders, including anxiety and depression.

Key Benefits of Progesterone

1. Balances estrogen
2. Responsible for breast development
3. Helps regulate sleep and body temperature
4. Assists in bone formation
5. Maintains blood sugar levels

6. Supports the efficiency of our thyroid
7. Acts as a natural diuretic

Signs of Low Progesterone

1. Anxiety
2. Mid-sleep awakening/sleep disturbances
3. Shorter cycles
4. Breast tenderness
5. Night sweats/hot flashes
6. Migraines
7. PMS
8. Weight gain

Testosterone

Testosterone, which I call the prince of sex hormones, plays a crucial role in women. Produced primarily by the ovaries and adrenal glands, it is essential for women's health and well-being in various ways.

Testosterone helps regulate energy levels and reduces symptoms like irritability, depression, and anxiety. It can play a part in overall mental well-being, impacting the function of neurotransmitters, including dopamine and serotonin. If levels are low, we can experience fatigue and a general lack of energy. Testosterone is also a key factor in sexual arousal, responsiveness, and satisfaction. There is limited research in the area of immunity, but some studies suggest that testosterone may help modulate immune responses, potentially offering protective effects against excessive inflammation.

Testosterone, along with estrogen, supports bone density. Adequate levels help prevent osteoporosis and bone fractures, especially as women age. As testosterone levels decline, bone and skeletal health are at risk. Similarly, although at one tenth of the levels of men, it contributes to our muscle maintenance and physical strength and plays a vital role in preserving lean muscle mass and regulating fat distribution. Lower testosterone can lead to a decrease in muscle mass, which can affect metabolism, weight maintenance, and body composition. Testosterone also has been found to support cognitive functions such as memory, spatial ability, and verbal fluency. Some studies suggest that testosterone levels impact brain health and may reduce the risk of cognitive decline and age-related mental disorders.

While the relationship between estrogen and the gut microbiome during menopause has been more extensively studied, research focusing on testosterone and the gut is limited. But we do know:

- In most menopausal women, testosterone levels are decreased, and this decrease is more important during the first years after menopause.
- There is a relationship between fat mass, fat distribution, and free-testosterone levels, especially in menopausal females. This contributes to body composition changes in the menopausal transition.
- There is a possible link between testosterone and the increase of visceral fat during menopause, which puts us at greatest risk for poor metabolic health, including diabetes and heart disease.

Key Benefits of Testosterone

1. Builds bones
2. Maintains muscle mass
3. Helps burn fat
4. Keeps energy levels high
5. Helps maintain memory
6. Increases your sense of emotional well-being, self-confidence, and motivation

Signs of Low Testosterone

1. Harder time building muscle
2. Poor blood sugar control
3. Low libido
4. Low motivation or mood

Non-Sex Hormones

You know, it's not all about sex, right? We have about fifty different hormones in our body, but here are some key ones that we need to keep in mind as we age.

The Thyroid and T4 and T3 Hormones

The thyroid—the butterfly-shaped gland in the front of our necks—is a major player when it comes to hormonal health because it orchestrates cellular functions and metabolism. This gland produces two hormones, T4 (thyroxine) and T3 (triiodothyronine), that support the function of the mitochondria, regulate metabolic rate and energy, control our weight, govern the metabolism of macros (protein, fat, and carbs), help with tissue repair and development, and regulate our menstrual cycles until we go into perimenopause and menopause. And you know what is coming next: With the changes and shifts in sex hormones, our thyroid function is altered. Remember our discussion about why women are more susceptible to autoimmune disorders? Well, I see many women at this stage of their lives developing what I affectionately call the "thyroid pause," or Hashimoto's thyroiditis, the most common manifestation of an underactive thyroid. This is when our immune system actually attacks our thyroid gland, creating a lot of inflammation. An underactive thyroid (as in Hashimoto's) is much more common than an overactive thyroid (as in Graves' disease).

Benefits of Thyroid Hormone

1. Increases the basal metabolic rate
2. Depending on the metabolic status, can help break down fats and increase LDL receptors in our liver
3. Stimulates the metabolism of carbohydrates
4. Anabolism of proteins; can also induce the breakdown of proteins in high doses
5. Allows the body to become more sensitive to the effects of catecholamines (epinephrine, norepinephrine)
6. Can affect mood
7. Affects fertility, ovulation, and menstruation

Signs of Underactive Thyroid Function (More Common)

1. Slow heart rate/bradycardia
2. Cold intolerance
3. Weight gain
4. Hair loss
5. Dry skin
6. Constipation
7. Fatigue
8. Hoarse voice
9. Changes in menstrual cycle, infertility
10. Goiter
11. Depression
12. Low libido
13. Changes in cognition, impaired memory or concentration

Signs of Overactive Thyroid Function

1. Elevated heart rate/tachycardia, palpitations
2. Heat intolerance, sweating
3. Weight loss
4. Greasy hair
5. Moist or sweaty skin
6. Diarrhea
7. Hyperactivity, tremors
8. Changes in menstrual cycle
9. Mania
10. Weakness, fatigue
11. Insomnia

Insulin

Secreted by the pancreas, this hormone plays an important role in blood glucose regulation, metabolism, cell growth and repair, brain function, and weight control. And don't think this gets off scot-free during perimenopause and menopause. Because of the changes in our sex hormones, we begin losing skeletal muscle mass, which translates into a negative impact on our insulin sensitivity. If we are still eating as we did at age eighteen (pizza for breakfast, chips, and soda), this may contribute to further loss of insulin sensitivity.

Benefits of Insulin

1. Maintains blood glucose levels
2. Supports a healthy metabolism
3. Provides cell growth and repair

4. Improves brain function
5. Weight control

Signs of Insulin Resistance

1. Skin tags
2. Acne
3. Weight gain
4. Headaches
5. Dizziness
6. Sleep disturbances
7. Elevated triglycerides
8. Elevated glucose, insulin, uric acid
9. Fatigue after meals
10. Craving sweets
11. Hair loss
12. NAFLD (nonalcoholic fatty liver disease)
13. PCOS
14. Gout
15. Cognitive changes: brain fog, etc.

THE ADRENAL GLANDS

The adrenal glands are endocrine glands that sit atop each kidney and produce hormones essential for the circadian rhythm, energy metabolism, blood pressure, and the body's stress response. They are part of the hypothalamic–pituitary–adrenal (HPA) axis.

The HPA axis is the communication axis between your brain and adrenals. The brain interprets environmental cues and signals the adrenals to produce stress hormones (epinephrine, norepinephrine, and cortisol) in the fight-or-flight response. This hormone cascade leads to physical changes, like increased blood sugar for energy, that allow you to run or fight danger. After the stress has subsided, the system returns to normal (what we call homeostasis).

Cortisol

I mentioned cortisol earlier in the book, because this fight-or-flight hormone response system is so key to our overall health and well-being. It prepares us for stress, acts as a natural anti-inflammatory agent, stimulates the immune system, boosts concentration, regulates appetite and cravings, and helps muscles respond to exercise. When we enter perimenopause/menopause, we produce less progesterone (our bodies' natural antianxiety hormone) and become less stress-resilient. With all the reports about how bad chronic stress is for our body, it should not come as a surprise to find out how this over-activation puts us into a sympathetic-dominant (fight-or-flight) state; impacts our insulin, oxytocin, and sex hormones; and can lead to chronic inflammation, lowered immunity and libido, and digestive distress. Excess cortisol also contributes to the dreaded cortisol belly and weight-loss resistance.

Christy could be a poster child for the perimenopausal stressed-out woman. As part of the "sandwich" generation, with aging parents, teenagers, and a busy career, she often felt like she never got a reprieve from taking care of everyone else in her life. When her father was hospitalized, critically, she felt like her stress levels had hit a wall. She was no longer sleeping well, she complained of daily headaches, she was craving sweets, and her pants felt tight.

Worried that she was at the point of no return, she came to see me. We made quick, simple edits to her daily schedule, adding ten minutes of light exposure in the morning, incorporating more protein at each meal, limiting caffeine, and incorporating adaptogenic herbs into her morning supplements and myo-inositol at night to help buffer cortisol. And we created a basic nighttime routine of putting her legs up the wall and doing five minutes of breathwork. Within several days, she felt less stress and more peace and calm. She continued these practices to keep the cortisol at bay. Thankfully, her father had an incredible recovery, which I suspect helped enormously.

Key Benefits of Cortisol

1. Acts as a natural anti-inflammatory if your body is impacted by injury, arthritis, or allergies
2. Stimulates the immune system
3. Boosts alertness, concentration, mood, and other cognitive functions
4. Regulates appetite and fights cravings
5. Maintains cardiovascular health
6. Aids in fertility
7. Helps muscles respond to exercise

Signs of Dysregulated Cortisol

1. Headaches
2. Weight gain, especially around the abdomen
3. Fatigue
4. Salt or sugar cravings
5. Low libido
6. Changes in menstrual cycle, infertility
7. Trouble concentrating, brain fog
8. Depression, irritability
9. Insomnia
10. Insulin resistance
11. Lowered immunity
12. Diarrhea or constipation, bloating

There is a popular term that speaks to the plight of a woman's life: "womb to tomb," the philosophy that women are regulated their entire lives by the reproductive endocrine system. In the following chapters, I'll help you figure out that this certainly does not have to be a life sentence as our natural hormones decline. We have powerful tools, including nutrition and lifestyle changes, targeted supplementation, and hormone replacement therapy.

Indeed, the regulation of hormones is critical to every essential system in our bodies, including the structure by which we stand, walk, and run: our bones. Let's take a look at the critical and often under-discussed effects of menopause on our bone health.

Chapter Summary

1. The predominant form of estrogen our bodies make prior to menopause is estradiol (E2); after menopause, our bodies make a weaker form of estrogen called estrone (E1).
2. The greatest variability of estrogen levels is during perimenopause (20 to 30 percent higher than in the rest of our lives), which helps account for many of the symptoms we experience.
3. Our microbiome is governed by shifts in estrogen, as well as the impact of the estrobolome to help us break down our estrogen and eliminate it from the body in conjunction with the enzyme beta-glucuronidase.
4. It is important to understand the interplay between our other hormones, including progesterone, testosterone, thyroid, insulin, and cortisol, in the context of navigating changes in midlife.

References for this chapter can be found on my website: cynthiathurlow.com/themenopausegut-references

Chapter 5

"I Feel It in My Bones"

So many of us don't think about bone health . . . until we have to. But our bones are one of the most underrated parts of the body. The body's skeletal system keeps us upright and allows us to move while it holds our muscles and organs in place. And while most of us think of our bones as static, they are actually dynamic, living organs that change and adapt to our life stages and environment by altering their size, shape, and density as needed. But like everything else in our body, our bones are adversely affected by aging and menopause. And you guessed it by now: A healthy gut begets healthier bones!

Catherine didn't think too much about her bones until she broke her wrist at the age of forty-two. Running errands on a busy Saturday, she simply tripped and fell, fracturing her right wrist. Her orthopedic surgeon suggested a baseline DXA scan (a special test that can measure bone strength), which revealed low bone mass (osteopenia). Several years later, at age fifty, Catherine was at the tail end of perimenopause, nearly menopausal. When she came to me, we talked about her long history of oral contraceptive use and how she had been a yo-yo dieter who lost and gained the same twenty-plus pounds year after year. The combination of the onset of late perimenopause, weight fluctuation, and use of contraceptives can wreak havoc on a woman's skeletal system and make her more likely to be diagnosed with osteoporosis later in life. When Catherine and I discussed a plan going forward, she remarked on how little she knew about bone health.

Our bones are vital, especially as we age. Here are some startling statistics about us and our bones:

- Women typically hit 95 percent of their peak bone density by age seventeen but see it fully peak between twenty-five and thirty years old. After thirty, there's a gradual decline in natural bone mass. Genetics has a lot to do with this, but other lifestyle choices, like good nutrition, not smoking, and exercise, may also play a role in achieving that peak bone density.
- One in two women over age fifty will break a bone because of osteoporosis, according to Johns Hopkins University, compared with one in four men.
- A 2015 study published in the *Journal of Clinical Endocrinology and Metabolism* showed that women who have severe hot flashes and night sweats during menopause will experience more bone loss and are at higher risk for hip fractures than women with less severe symptoms.
- For women, the majority of bone loss happens in the first five to six years after their final period. They lose as much as 10 to 20 percent during that time. Women lose bone density twice as fast as men because, generally speaking, men have larger skeletons, and their bone loss doesn't accelerate like women's does. Their bone loss starts later, around age sixty-five.

Blame Estrogen Loss (Again)

How can we lose so much bone density? Easy answer: Because of that darn natural decline of estrogen during menopause. In addition to everything else you have read in this book thus far, estrogen helps protect our bones, strengthening them and preventing bone loss. Specifically, it helps maintain a healthy equilibrium between osteoblasts (cells that help build bone) and osteoclasts (cells that break down bone tissue to make room for new, healthier bone).

I often compare our skeletal system to a giant Lego tower. Two types of special workers in your body help take care of this tower. Osteoblasts are the builders; they add new Lego pieces to make the tower stronger and taller. Osteoclasts are the cleanup crew. They remove old or broken Lego pieces to make room for new ones. In a healthy body, these two teams work together—builders and cleanup crew balance each other out.

We always want to maintain healthy levels of estrogen that will protect bone by keeping this osteoblast-osteoclast equilibrium. Unfortunately, when we reach late perimenopause and menopause, estrogen levels decline, and so does the hormone's protective role in our bones, and we see that equilibrium teeter off balance. The cleanup crew of osteoclasts starts working too much, and the osteoblasts can't keep up with rebuilding. This can cause bones to weaken, like a Lego tower missing too many pieces.

The Gut Also Plays a Role

If you have been following along, the gut's role in our bone health should come as no surprise to you. Just like many parts of the body, studies reveal how our bones are affected by the gut, in particular by the directional communication loop between our gut, brain, and bones called the gut–bone–brain axis (GBA). Because of its impact on cortisol, gut hormones, and neurotransmitters, the gut microbiota is also considered a virtual endocrine "organ" (even though it's not an organ), with specific effects on bone metabolism. The connections are still being studied, but there are a few things we do know: The gut microbiota helps regulate bone growth and bone strength, as well as bone loss and fracture risk, by influencing activity and function of osteoblasts and osteoclasts. Recent studies have shown that our gut microbiota does this through the immune system. The endocrine system is at work, too, with insulin-like growth factor 1 (IGF-1), which can also promote the differentiation and growth of bone cells, including osteoblasts, osteoclasts, and chondrocytes (cartilage cells that maintain the collagen matrix), and enhance normal interactions among them. This newly discovered close interrelationship has led the medical community to study *osteoimmunology*, a big fancy word for the study of how bone health and metabolism are intricately linked to our immune system.

As you have read, gut bacteria help the immune system to stay calm and not overreact. And that calm immune system helps bones stay strong. When we go through menopause, the depleted estrogen disrupts our gut bacteria balance, and the immune system gets out of balance as well. An overactive immune system can send messages that make osteoclasts work too much, breaking down bones faster than they can be rebuilt. (The imbalance between progesterone and estrogen continues to drive excess bone breakdown in menopause; it is debated whether it is primarily driven by estrogen or by this imbalance.)

The double whammy is that estrogen deficiency in menopause alters intestinal microbial composition and structure, leading to decreased microbial diversity. This means the loss of estrogen has an enormous impact on the types of bacteria helpers we have as well as the diversity of our bacteria—both being bad for our bone health. One study showed decreased bacterial richness and diversity and significant changes in the gut microbial community in postmenopausal osteoporosis, indicating a strong connection between bone and microbiome.

Leaky Gut Impacts Bone Health

The small intestine (SI) comes into play here, as it contains 80 percent of our immune cells (along with our large intestine), and immune regulation plays a significant role in the overall regulation of bone metabolism. Any decrease in estrogen increases the permeability of the outermost epithelial layer of the SI (a.k.a. leaky gut) and may enhance the levels of bone breakdown and inflammation. Research suggests that any breach in the lining of the SI has the potential to negatively impact bone health. Again, this speaks to the significant role that our sex hormones play in maintaining the tightness of the lining of our small intestine, which when breached can create low-grade inflammation. This inflammation in the intestines might negatively impact the absorption of minerals like calcium and reduce circulating levels of fat-soluble vitamins, like D and K, thus reducing bone mass.

Recent studies have demonstrated a close relationship between the intestinal microbiota and bone metabolism, providing evidence that the intestinal microbiome may serve as a good therapeutic tool for the treatment of postmenopausal osteoarthritis (PMO).

What We Need to Watch Out for as Our Bones Age

Bottom line? As we age and estrogen levels decline, we have to be ever more diligent about our bone health, as not only are our bones less dense as we age, but they take longer to heal. If we don't find ways to keep those osteoblasts and osteoclasts working, we risk getting the following conditions:

Osteopenia: Often thought of as the precursor to osteoporosis, this is simply low bone density. It does not require intervention, per se, but you'll need to be aware of what contributes to lower bone mass at younger ages in order to proactively address it with lifestyle measures. Genetics plays an important role in a person's bone mineral density, and Caucasian and Asian women with petite body types are at the highest risk of osteopenia. Many of us who took oral contraceptives throughout our teens, twenties, and thirties missed out on the peak bone- and muscle-mass-building years and are high-risk (like Catherine). I, in fact, have been osteopenic intermittently for the past ten to fifteen years. I share this as a cautionary tale because, like many women, I thought I was doing all the right things, but lifestyle does play a huge role.

Osteoporosis: Literally meaning "porous bone," this is a serious condition characterized by either insufficient bone formation, excessive bone loss, or a combination of the two. It leads to an increased risk for fractures, particularly of the hip, spine, and wrist. Osteoporosis impacts forty-four million Americans and more than 150 million people worldwide—that's a staggering number of people who are walking around with poor bone health.

The first five years of menopause is when we're at most significant risk for osteoporosis and potential fractures. Another sobering thought: Hip and vertebral fractures may shorten life expectancy. The mortality rate within one year of long-term bedridden patients is 20 percent, and the permanent disability rate is 50 percent.

Assessing Your Bone Health

How do we know our bones are heading down this path? Healthcare providers use an X-ray-type machine called the dual-energy X-ray absorptiometry (DXA) scan, which measures your bone mineral density. Its T-score shows how much your bone mass differs from the bone mass of an average healthy thirty-year-old. A score of 0 or somewhere between +1 and –1 is considered normal and healthy. If the score is –1 to –2.4, that's considered osteopenia. A score of –2.5 or lower signals osteoporosis. The higher that negative number becomes, the more severe the osteoporosis. Some people can acquire osteoporosis early, but most cases are postmenopausal osteoporosis. PMO is an estrogen-deficiency-induced metabolic bone disorder characterized by reduced bone mass and structural changes that increase the risk of bone fragility and susceptibility to fracture in postmenopausal women. And—what I find most frightening, both as a middle-aged woman and as a nurse practitioner—is that the CDC guidelines are for women to be screened starting at the age of *sixty-five*, and for women aged fifty to sixty-four *only* if they have had a family member with a fracture. This is far too late to intervene—women should be screened and have had discussions about bone health much earlier in life. Personally, I wish all women were screened in their thirties, especially after pregnancy or lactation.

Unfortunately, osteoporosis is usually not detected until you sustain your first fracture (like Catherine), and because of that, it is often called a silent disease. Nevertheless, the condition can cause back pain, loss of height over time, and a stooped posture, which is called kyphosis.

Other Hormones That Come into Play

It is not just estrogen that impacts bones and the gut microbiome. Other hormones, including androgens, progesterone, and even cortisol, play a small role in bone health throughout our lives, especially during perimenopause and menopause. Bone growth, modeling, and remodeling are modulated by estrogen, androgen, and growth hormones, all of which decline with age.

Progesterone: There isn't a lot of research on the effects of progesterone on the bones, but here is what we do know: Progesterone is active in bone metabolism; it is women's bone-formation-stimulating hormone. It appears to act directly on bone by engaging osteoblasts, promoting bone formation and/or increasing bone turnover. Bone mineral density (BMD) loss is more rapid in perimenopause than after menopause; decreased bone formation due to progesterone deficiency contributes. Also, progesterone is estradiol's partner hormone in bone. It appears to play important roles in the achievement of an ideal, peak BMD in adolescence and young adulthood and in the prevention of bone loss during pre- and likely perimenopausal life phases, leading to a normal peak perimenopausal BMD.

SARCOPENIA AND MUSCULOSKELETAL SYNDROME OF MENOPAUSE (MSSM)

Sarcopenia is defined as muscle loss with aging. We may not even consider this normal trajectory in our muscular skeletal health . . . until it changes, seemingly right before our eyes. The musculoskeletal syndrome of menopause (MSSM) is a new syndrome coined by Dr. Vonda Wright to describe the umbrella of all the common musculoskeletal symptoms related to low estrogen, including joint, bone, and cartilage pain, sarcopenia, osteoporosis, reduced mobility and range of motion (ROM), and muscle pain.

Skeletal muscle loss begins at age 35, continuing at a rate of 1 to 2 percent every year. The muscle loss increases to 3 percent per year after age 65. Sarcopenia is not just a change in body composition, it's a disorder that increases our chances of falls, fractures, and eventual disability. This is where lifestyle measures, including maintaining a healthy microbiome, strength training, flexibility and balance training, HRT, and targeted nutrition and testing are essential for optimal living. Current risk factors for sarcopenia include: low protein intake, low vitamin D intake, low physical activity, and hormonal changes occurring during perimenopause and menopause.

Sarcopenia is sneaky. Kelly was in late perimenopause when she felt the shift in her body composition. She noticed more body fat in the familiar places—hips, thighs, buttocks—despite keeping up with cardiovascular exercise and eating a healthy amount of solid macros. She was already quite lean, so she was readily observant of changes to her body.

Previously, she had done fitness competitions; she estimated her body fat percentage in the 15 percent range for most of her thirties. We did a bioimpedance measurement and her fat-free mass was in the high twenties with no other changes to her lifestyle, and her lean body mass (muscle) was reduced by 20 percent.

She was stunned. We swapped strength training for the cardio exercise and increased her protein, ensured that her sleep and stress were dialed in, and added in creatine monohydrate. We tested her hormones and noted that her progesterone, estrogen, and testosterone were all low, so we added in HRT as well. Within three months she had lost body fat and felt "more toned." It takes time to build muscle in middle age, but she was well on her way to getting back to fighting form.

Testosterone: As with progesterone, there is little information on the effects of testosterone on bone health, but here is what we *do* know: Both estrogen and androgens inhibit bone resorption. Testosterone aids in bone growth, as it acts directly on osteoblasts and indirectly impacts bone growth through its effects on growth factors and cytokines. As we age, lowered levels of testosterone may seriously affect bone health. However, research is inconclusive and limited with regard to women.

Cortisol: The fight-or-flight hormone plays a part in our bone health as well. High levels of cortisol both increase bone resorption (through inhibiting calcium absorption) and halt bone formation by inhibiting osteoblast effects. Cortisol may negatively affect bone density by altering bone turnover, impairing intestinal absorption and renal reabsorption of calcium, and, in perimenopausal women, by inhibiting reproductive hormones. Yet more reasons to control your stress and be proactive at this stage of life.

Other Risk Factors That Can Affect Bone Health

While heredity can be a big factor, bone fragility can be mitigated with the right lifestyle changes. Here are the usual suspects:

Nutrition: No bones about it, nutrition has a crucial impact on osteoporosis. Low-protein diets, low calcium intake through food, vitamin D and K deficiencies, high phosphorus levels, ultraprocessed foods, heavy alcohol consumption, and soda consumption are all universally considered risk factors for osteoporosis.

Unfortunately, the Standard American Diet, which is full of ultraprocessed foods—highly palatable but high in calories and full of inflammatory seed oils, refined carbs, and sugars—is still the mainstay of most of the US. Seventy percent of Americans consume the bulk of their food intake from ultraprocessed foods. Long-term consumption of SAD could result in a decrease in the diversity of the gut microbiota and promote inflammation, which can lead to digestive disorders, damage to the intestinal lining (and thus leaky gut), and leakage of toxic bacterial metabolites into the circulatory system, all of which may result in the progression of systemic low-grade inflammation, which then contributes to the development of poor bone health and potentially osteoporosis.

Impact of stress: Chronic stress causes endocrine system dysregulation and can disrupt bone homeostasis. We become less stress-resilient in perimenopause and menopause, which creates a vicious cycle. Add in low estrogen and it is the perfect storm for bone breakdown.

When that stress hormone cortisol kicks in, it can disrupt the structural integrity of the gut lining and contribute to a weakened microbiome, further depleting bone health. One study shows that low-grade inflammation and hyper-activation of the sympathetic nervous system during psychological stress can be detrimental to bone health; several other studies have demonstrated that psychological stress is associated with osteoporosis. Bottom line? Stress begets leaky gut begets bone loss.

Oral contraceptives (OCs) and Depo-Provera (DMPA): I imagine that many women reading this book are of a generation who were prescribed OCs in our teens through our thirties and had no idea this would contribute to so many risk factors. Many women from my generation were immensely impacted by the start of OCs as teens into their twenties, when the impact on bone health was catastrophic. But here we are, so let's get down to it so we can do something about it.

Oral contraceptives are synthetic hormones designed to suppress ovulation. According to Dr. Felice Gersh, OCs increase blood pressure and blood-clotting risks, are pro-inflammatory, change the composition of the microbiome, and impact breast cancer risk. Here's more about their impact on bone health:

- OC use seems to be most impactful on younger women, especially teens: Studies have shown contraceptives can compromise teenagers' bone mineral acquisition, especially within three years of starting menstruation. Contraception is commonly prescribed to adolescents for many reasons, including pregnancy prevention, treatment for acne, and to ease painful periods. Although the use of these hormones generally has no effect or benefits on bone health in mature, perimenopausal women, the same may not be true for adolescents. The teen years are a critical period for acquiring peak bone strength: 90 to 95 percent of bone mass in women is achieved by age eighteen. This is a big reason why younger women are more impacted by contraception than older women. It's not known if the loss is fully reversible after stopping OCs or if their use results in lifelong compromised bone strength.

A 2013 comprehensive study showed that women taking a combined oral contraceptive (progesterone and estrogen) had a nearly 50 percent increased risk of developing inflammatory bowel disease. The study also showed that OCs could increase the risk of Crohn's disease threefold in women with a family history of the disease.

Depo-Provera (medroxyprogesterone acetate), which is an injectable contraceptive, has significant side effects as well. It's part of a class of drugs called long-acting reversible contraceptives (LARCs). It prevents ovulation and thickens cervical mucus, making the uterus less hospitable for a fertilized egg to implant. Women typically receive an intramuscular injection every twelve weeks to prevent pregnancy. Side effects can include weight gain, headaches, bone loss, and more.

- Research shows that DMPA use for twelve months is associated with a loss of bone mineral density; mean bone loss in DMPA users was 2.74 percent.
- The Food and Drug Administration (FDA) added a black-box warning to DMPA packaging in 2004 cautioning against long-term use (more than two years), as bone loss may be quite substantial. On a positive note, the literature shows the decrease in bone mineral density in users of DMPA to be reversible once its use has stopped.

To be clear, reliable contraception is important, but there should be explicit, deliberate explanations of the long-term consequences of using these options, including changes to the gut microbiome and the impact on bone health. Overall, the skeletal effects of some forms of hormonal contraception have a greater impact on adolescent females than on mature women.

All this research is stark in its findings and makes one big point: The concept of fully informed consent is critically important for *all* women.

How to Mitigate Bone Loss

We'll get more detailed in part 2, but here are some key takeaways to remember for staving off bone loss:

- Be physically active. Progressive weight-bearing exercises such as lifting light weights, and high-intensity interval training (HIIT) or sprint interval training (SIT) will help stimulate bone activity.
- Reconsider your oral contraceptive options sooner rather than later; this is even more important for younger women. Again, fully informed consent about the long-term implications of the choices we make is important.
- Maintaining a healthy weight is important. Consume adequate protein, which is approximately thirty to fifty grams per meal. Don't chronically eat in a caloric deficit or yo-yo diet. Eat calcium-rich foods and plenty of fiber. Think dark leafy greens, sweet potatoes, fatty fish, and citrus fruits. Avoid alcohol consumption. Do not smoke. If you do, quit. Now.
- Hormone replacement therapy is worth discussing with your ob-gyn, internist, or hormone-savvy provider.

Our gut, hormones, immune system, and bone health in perimenopause and menopause are all connected—and complicated. What you just read was a mini medical school semester in menopausal health. You have learned a lot about how the body changes—and also ways we can mitigate those changes. Now, are you ready to put it into action?

Chapter Summary

1. Consider your choices of contraception—when you start them and how they can impact the trajectory of your bone health long term.
2. Start prioritizing strength training *now*, so that you can build solid habits for the rest of your life.
3. Factor in dietary choices now that support a healthy microbiome and bone health.
4. Don't smoke and don't drink excessively.

References for this chapter can be found on my website: cynthiathurlow.com/themenopausegut-references

Part 2

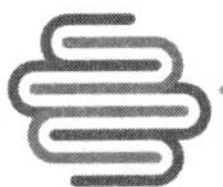

The Menopause Gut Plan

Menopause is inevitable. Suffering through it is not. There is much we can do to mitigate the onslaught of changes our body experiences, and this plan is your road map to do just that. It includes a comprehensive look at how our lifestyle and nutrition choices are crucial in managing our health from perimenopause through postmenopause.

The way I see it (and I have seen it with my patients and clients), there are many important components that will help you thrive and not just survive the transition from perimenopause into menopause: nutrition, exercise, sleep, and stress management. I'll also give you information on treatments that go beyond what we can do on our own, and that includes targeted testing, supplementation, and, when appropriate, HRT and other prescription medications. I also include a starter kit of nutritious—and delicious!—recipes to help you on the road to a more healthy and energized life.

Ready to feel better?

Chapter 6

Nutrition Is Your Ammunition

Jennifer was fifty-five and super busy. She was a marketing executive at a food-based company, and because she'd waited to have kids until a bit later in life, she was still shuttling around two middle schoolers to various activities. The demands of being a working mom of tweens made her tired. It didn't help that her digestive system seemed to be working against her, and she was constipated and bloated. She had gained weight around the middle and lost her waist, which she attributed to not exercising and bingeing on hyper-palatable foods, which she called "stress eating." Being menopausal just. Made. Everything. Worse.

Like Jennifer, many women complain about the stubborn weight that seems to just appear as we get older. It's not simply anecdotal: Menopause is associated with an increased prevalence of weight gain and obesity. And no matter what the weight-loss trends are—whether it's a GLP-1 drug, like Ozempic, or the latest fad diet—losing weight and being healthy always comes down to basics. And of course, hormones play a huge role here, and that's what gets confusing: All the strategies that worked before no longer do. The interrelationship between our dietary choices and how we feel is crucial because after all, food is how we provide our bodies with energy to function. We may have gotten away with eating McDonald's and Doritos when we indulged in our twenties, but as we get older, our bodies become less forgiving. In perimenopause and menopause, the food choices we make become even more important. In this chapter, I want to show you how you can better support your body with the right nutrition to lessen the likelihood you will experience most of the worst perimenopause and menopause symptoms, as well as increase your energy and help support your immune system.

There is substantial evidence that perimenopause is associated with a more rapid increase in fat mass, redistribution of fat to the abdomen, and an increase in total body fat. After menopause, there is a clear increase in body fat and a decrease in lean muscle mass. It is probably one of the more demoralizing consequences of the menopausal transition: We can no longer fit into our favorite clothes that we looked so good in during our thirties, and we may start to worry about changes in body composition. The fluctuating and then declining estrogen levels and changes in insulin sensitivity lead to a shift in fat distribution, causing more fat to accumulate around our abdomens—known as visceral fat. Unlike subcutaneous fat, which sits just under the skin, visceral fat surrounds vital organs like the liver, pancreas, and intestines, making it much more harmful to overall health. Visceral fat leads to an increased risk of heart disease (the number one killer of women), diabetes, poor metabolic health, strokes, fatty liver disease, neurocognitive decline, and chronic inflammation. This type of fat is pathogenic and harmful and should be avoided. In fact, we want to avoid gaining visceral fat like our lives are dependent on it.

One of the ways to address this is by changing how we approach nutrition and meal frequency.

A Healthy Diet for a Healthy Microbiome

The gut microbiome's diversity is ever more important as we transition into menopause. The number one priority is how to make our gut as diverse and rich as possible so it can maximize its efforts in all areas of our body, including fighting inflammation, improving our immune system, supporting a healthy metabolism, and maintaining a healthy weight (and limiting or avoiding the accumulation of visceral fat). That seems like a great deal to consider, doesn't it? But if you stick to a simple, sustainable list, it will be relatively easy to follow. You want a diet rich in macronutrients (that's protein, fat, and carbs), as well as fiber, the trifecta of pro-, pre-, and postbiotics, polyphenols, signaling molecules (What the heck are they? Read on. . . .), and water. Lots of it.

Macronutrients

There are three main macros that make up the substantive part of our diet: protein, carbs, and fats. All three strongly influence the gut microbiome and can impact our health substantially.

Protein

Protein, which breaks down into amino acids, is a building block of hormones. It helps to create hormones that support growth and the production of neurotransmitters. It keeps our energy levels balanced by keeping our blood sugar stable, which in turn keeps our energy stable. It also strengthens immunity, supports lean muscle mass, and promotes bone health. Need I say more?

As we age, our protein requirements increase because our skeletal muscles require more stimulus to grow, both from adequate protein intake and from strength training. It is important to both grow *and* maintain our muscle as we age, because when we lose muscle mass, we are more likely to become insulin resistant. It is not just about body composition; it is about our metabolic health.

There's an important theory surrounding protein called the protein leverage hypothesis (PLH). It suggests that humans have a strong biological drive to consume a certain amount of protein, and when diets are low in this macro, we'll eat more total calories to compensate. This can lead to overeating and obesity. Protein is one of the most important fuels for your body; it helps your muscles grow, keeps your brain sharp, and makes you feel full. If you don't eat enough protein, your body tells you, "I'm still hungry! Eat more food!" So, you might eat chips, cookies, or other snacks, trying to feel full. But if those foods don't have enough protein, your body keeps asking for more. This can lead to overeating and weight gain.

If you eat enough protein-rich foods like beef, eggs, chicken, fish, beans, and nuts, your body feels satisfied sooner, and you don't overeat. I have my patients aim for thirty to fifty grams of protein per meal—this helps keep them satiated and helps them avoid late-night bingeing. If you have a higher protein intake, then you will be preserving and building lean mass and facilitating body fat loss. Whereas if you don't eat enough protein and you're trying to restrict calories, lean mass is the first thing that goes.

Bottom line: We need more protein with aging, not less—and the sooner we can build and maintain our muscle, the healthier and more active we will be.

Overall, evolving evidence supports the concept that lean body mass can be better maintained if protein is consumed at a level higher than the Recommended Daily Allowance (RDA), which is only 0.36 grams per pound of body weight. I think the RDA's recommendations are just sufficient to keep you alive; they are not optimal recommendations. My recommendation is:

Daily intake goal: 30–50 grams per meal

Power foods: Beef, bison, elk, wild boar, chicken, turkey, and duck; fatty fish, like SMASH (salmon, mackerel, anchovies, sardines, and herring); tuna, cod, flounder, mahi-mahi, trout, and grouper; shrimp, lobster, clams, mussels, crab, oysters, scallops, and squid; eggs; and plant-based proteins: legumes, beans, nuts, and seeds, like chia and flax; quinoa and ancient grains, like amaranth, millet, and buckwheat; and fermented soy.

Dairy sources: Full-fat Greek yogurt, full-fat cottage cheese, raw-milk cheese, and kefir (both fermented food and dairy) are all reasonable options for getting more protein into your diet.

Now, I'm a realist and understand that sometimes protein powders and bars can be a way to attain our protein goals on busy days. If you tolerate dairy, a clean whey protein (short ingredient list, no artificial sugars, etc.) is a nice option for when your protein macros fall short. There are few, if any, protein bars that aren't glorified candy bars, but I do find beef, venison, or bison jerky is a nice way to have protein on the go. Remember to check those food labels to avoid junky ingredients (such as seed oils and artificial sweeteners).

THE ANIMAL VS. PLANT-BASED DEBATE

If you don't eat enough protein, you will get energy from fats and carbs. Many people differ on where we should get most of our protein from—there are pros and cons to both animal (meat, eggs, dairy, fish) and plant-based protein (beans, lentils, quinoa). See the following and you can decide for yourself.

Pros of Animal-Based Protein:

- Contains all essential amino acids in the right proportions, which is crucial for muscle maintenance, growth, and repair.
- Has higher levels of leucine, a key amino acid for muscle protein synthesis that can help prevent muscle loss (sarcopenia), which accelerates in the perimenopause-to-menopause transition.
- Has key nutrients that plant-based proteins typically lack: zinc, iron, vitamin B_{12}, selenium, and phosphorus.
- Provides calcium, vitamin D, and collagen to support bone density and reduce the risk of osteoporosis.
- Contains heme iron, a form of iron that's a key component of hemoglobin, a protein in red blood cells that carries oxygen throughout the body. It's more easily absorbed than non-heme iron (found in plant foods), reducing the risk of anemia.

Cons:

- Can run up your grocery bill; however, there are ways to obtain animal-based proteins more inexpensively through stores such as Aldi, Costco, and Trader Joe's, which often have wild-caught, pasture-raised, and even grass-fed animal-based protein at more affordable prices. Another way is to purchase directly from farmers or buy cow shares. Purchase the best quality that your budget permits. That includes wild-caught fish, pasture-raised chicken and pork, and grass-fed beef.

- May have higher amounts of fat and cholesterol. If you are trying to lose weight, choosing leaner cuts of meat, poultry, and fish is important.
- Some women don't tolerate fatty cuts of meat, poultry, and fish as well as others. Personally, I do best with leaner protein choices, but I have plenty of friends and colleagues who can tolerate higher-fat versions.

Pros of Plant-Based Protein:

- Rich in fiber and antioxidants, supports gut microbiome balance, which plays a role in hormone regulation. Adequate fiber intake is a struggle for many of my female patients and clients because we tend to eat more processed foods that are devoid of fiber.
- Permits a variety of ethically conscious options.

Cons:

- Most plant proteins lack one or more essential amino acids; however, there are a few choices for complete plant-based proteins, like hemp seeds, chia seeds, spirulina, buckwheat, and soy.
- Many of the plant-based proteins are high in carbohydrates; I find that most middle-aged women need to watch their carb intake, even from healthy sources. The problem is that many of these proteins are too high in their carbohydrate-to-protein ratio. Example: 1 cup of quinoa is 8 grams of protein and 39 grams of carbs. That's totally unbalanced for most women. I typically suggest 30 grams of carbs per meal. If someone is not metabolically healthy, they may benefit from limiting carbohydrate intake (but not excluding them entirely).

- Plant proteins are absorbed slightly less efficiently than animal proteins, requiring higher intake to meet protein needs.
- Plant-based diets often lack vitamin B_{12}, essential for energy and nerve function. Other missing nutrients can include: creatine, heme iron, taurine, docosahexaenoic acid (DHA), which is an omega-3 fatty acid, and vitamin D_3. (We will discuss supplements in greater detail in chapter 12.)
- There are concerns about soy, which constitutes a major protein source in plant-based diets. Soybean plants are largely genetically modified (GMOs), and long-term exposure to GMOs can be detrimental to our health. Some examples of soy are tofu, edamame, and many vegan protein powders and bars. I generally caution my patients about consuming soy, unless it is fermented like miso or natto.

My takeaway: I personally do best with an animal-based diet, but I will add lentils or beans to a salad, as well as have miso soup and occasionally small portions of nuts and seeds. A balanced mix of plant and animal proteins can offer muscle and bone support, heart health, and hormone balance during the perimenopause-to-menopause transition. If you choose the plant-based protein path, be even more mindful about getting sufficient protein to retain good metabolic health and body composition. Prioritize complete proteins (spirulina, buckwheat, hemp seeds, fermented soy, and chia). Be conscientious about balancing protein intake with carbohydrate intake, especially if you are not metabolically healthy, and consider supplementation with options like creatine monohydrate, B_{12}, and other supplements to fill nutritional gaps.

Fat

We are talking good fats here. This macro is instrumental in supporting a healthy blood sugar, helping with absorption of fat-soluble vitamins like A, D, E, and K, and supporting the composition of our cellular membranes.

It also helps support growth and development, provides energy, helps with satiety (feel full longer!), and enhances the flavor of food.

Fats are classified based on their *saturation*, a term that refers to the number of hydrogen atoms in their chains of fatty acids. When a fatty acid carries the maximum number of hydrogen atoms, it is said to be saturated. The more saturated a fat is, the more stable it is at room temperature. Examples are beef, dairy products, butter, and some vegetables, like coconut. If there are one or more places on the chain where hydrogens are missing, the fatty acid is considered unsaturated. These are divided into monounsaturated and polyunsaturated. Monounsaturated fats are found in foods like olives, olive oil, avocados, avocado oil, nuts, and seeds. Polyunsaturated fats are found in walnuts, flaxseed, and salmon and can be further divided into omega-3 and omega-6 fatty acids.

NOT ALL FAT IS BAD

By the way, saturated fats and cholesterol are not inherently bad. What's that? Saturated fats aren't all that bad, according to new research. Considering we have been hearing how saturated fats can lead to heart disease for nearly sixty years, that may come as a big surprise. But recently there has been pushback on this standard theory of the diet-heart hypothesis. There have been more than twenty papers that have "largely concluded that saturated fats have no effect on cardiovascular disease, cardiovascular mortality or total mortalities," according to science writer Nina Teicholz, who goes on to assert that the studies suggesting saturated fat causes heart disease were based on "weak, associational evidence." And I believe our current dietary guidelines should be updated to reflect this research.

Choose foods with "good" healthy fats and avoid unhealthy polyunsaturated fats (like soybean, canola, cottonseed, sunflower, safflower, and seed oils) that are highly adulterated and rancid or exposed to toxic solvents. Also avoid trans fats, which are outlawed in the US. "Good" unsaturated fats—monounsaturated and polyunsaturated fats—reduce disease risk.

If you already have fat in your protein, there's no need to add it in the meal; if your meal has a leaner protein, you can safely add in some fats. (Example: rib-eye steak vs. filet mignon; duck breast vs. chicken breast; salmon vs. cod fillet). Be mindful of portions; fats are 9 calories per gram versus 4 calories per gram for protein and carbs; they add up fast! Measure your portions if you are unsure.

Tip: Although I am not a proponent of tracking calories, it can be helpful to understand what a proper portion of olive oil is (one to two tablespoons) to help avoid unnecessarily large portions that can contribute to weight-loss resistance over time.

PROTEIN THAT PACKS A PUNCH

You don't have to make big, sweeping changes to your daily diet to move the needle on your gut health. Just a few tweaks can make a real difference. One thing I do to get extra protein is make it a topping: Add beans or lentils to soups or salads, sprinkle nuts or seeds on salads or vegetable dishes, swap crunchy cheese like Whisps for croutons, or mix Greek yogurt with lemon or lime and garlic powder and drizzle it over tacos or fajitas.

Another way to sneak in protein is when making dips (a great way to eat more vegetables), use Greek yogurt or cottage cheese as a base, and try one of these tasty ideas:

- Mix in ranch or taco seasoning.
- Fold in Buffalo sauce and chopped rotisserie chicken (perfect for game days).
- Blend with any fresh herbs you have on hand and some chopped English cucumber. Thin your dip with a little water and it makes a tasty salad dressing.

- Craving a sweet treat? Blend cottage cheese with unsweetened cocoa powder and a few dates until smooth; dip in apple wedges or strawberries.

Carbohydrates

Carbs have been demonized for far too long. Some will claim carbs are the root of all health issues; I prefer to take each patient as their own individual and determine their threshold of carb tolerance. But the truth is, whole, nutrient-dense carbs are healthy, and processed varieties are not. How to tell the difference? Well, if it is in a box, bag, or can or if it has a long list of ingredients that you cannot pronounce, it is probably processed.

There are two main categories of carbs:

1. **Refined (or simple) carbs** are short molecule chains. Simple carbs are easy for your body to break down. As the name suggests, they have a very basic chemical structure. They may be monosaccharides comprising a single sugar molecule, like glucose, or they may be disaccharides, which have two simple sugars linked together. Examples are table sugar (sucrose), jam, candy, syrup, and processed foods.

2. **Whole (or complex) carbs,** a.k.a. starches, are made of multiple sugar molecules, which eventually get broken down into glucose during digestion. These are called oligosaccharides and polysaccharides. Complex carbs take longer to digest than simple carbs do. This means they have a less immediate impact on blood sugar, causing it to rise more slowly. Portions are key; aim for servings of a quarter cup to a half cup per meal, and perhaps more on days when you are more active. Examples include beans, winter squash, potatoes, sweet potatoes, and ancient grains like amaranth, millet, spelt, and buckwheat.

An easy way to remember: Refined carbs have been processed, with the natural fiber and other nutrients removed or changed. Whole carbs are unprocessed, meaning they have not been refined in any way, and they contain the fiber found naturally in food.

Remember, as it pertains to overall carbs, be mindful of portions, especially if you have a significant amount of weight to lose, are insulin- or leptin-resistant, or are metabolically inflexible (prediabetic and insulin resistant).

Fiber

Fiber is a nondigestible, plant-based carbohydrate. It is naturally found in many fruits, vegetables, beans, nuts, grains, and seeds. You will want a lot of different kinds to help balance your hormones, support gut health, reduce inflammation, and boost your mood. There are many ways to get more fiber into our diets to support our microbiome.

Ideally, we want to aim for thirty plant varieties over the course of a week. There is a clear link between low fiber and lower microbial diversity that leads to obesity, so fiber is key to helping maintain a healthy weight. Some soluble fiber acts as a prebiotic; these include inulin and fructooligosaccharides, found in onions, leeks, garlic, asparagus, chicory root, and Jerusalem artichoke (a.k.a. fartichoke!).

While some people take powders, as with every other nutrient, it is really important to get fiber from real food, not commercial powder. There are two types:

Soluble fiber dissolves in water and slows down carbohydrate digestion, which can make you feel full longer and help stabilize blood sugar levels. Soluble fiber is found in foods like raspberries, pears, green peas, broccoli, quinoa, oats, lentils, and black beans.

Insoluble fiber doesn't break down in the digestive system, as it retains water, but it helps to move food through the digestive system (and therefore helps us poop better). Insoluble fiber is found in foods like nuts, seeds, fruits, vegetables, and some grains. Interestingly, a study of healthy individuals found that weight gain was inversely correlated with the consumption of dietary fiber over time, thus demonstrating that fiber has a role in limiting weight gain in the long term.

Daily intake goal: 20 to 25 grams. If you haven't had a lot of fiber in your diet before, go slowly to avoid digestive upset, gas, or bloating.

FODMAPs

Some women are sensitive to FODMAPs, a group of carbohydrates found in various foods that we eat. FODMAP is an acronym:

F: Fermentable

O: Oligosaccharides (fiber found in foods like onions, garlic, beans, and wheat)

D: Disaccharides (includes lactose, a commonly malabsorbed sugar found in dairy)

M: Monosaccharides (includes fructose, found in some fruits and processed foods)

P: Polyols (sugar alcohols added to sugar-free gum and candy and found naturally in some fruits and vegetables)

For some, these FODMAP foods are poorly absorbed in the small intestine, draw extra water from the intestines, and are rapidly fermented by gut bacteria, meaning they have the potential to cause or create GI distress, such as gas, bloating, diarrhea, and pain.

If you think you are sensitive to these foods, cut them out of your diet to see if there is any improvement.

OMEGA-3s:

We can't forget about these powerhouses. Omega-3s are essential fatty acids that your body needs; they are crucial for brain function, heart health, and reducing inflammation. Because we can only convert a small amount of ALA into EPA and DHA, most needs to come from our diets.

Types of Omega-3s:

1. **EPA (eicosapentaenoic acid):** Found in fatty fish, like salmon and mackerel.
2. **DHA (docosahexaenoic acid):** Also found in fish and other seafood.
3. **ALA (alpha-linolenic acid):** Found in ground flaxseed, walnuts, soybeans, and omega-3-rich eggs.

Tracking Your Macros

Finding it hard to keep track of what you are eating? There's a great free app, Cronometer, that helps you track all nutritional information. Track your macros for a week on Cronometer and see how you are doing day-to-day with your protein, fat, and carbohydrate intake; aim for two to three meals spaced out throughout the day.

How can I get all three macronutrients in my meals? Many of my clients ask me this very question. I always give them this general rule of thumb: By eating three vegetables to one piece of fruit, this keeps the emphasis on fiber and less on sweet fruits. (I find that most of my patients eat too much fruit and very few true vegetables.)

An example of a daily meal plan:

Breakfast: Omelet with a side of sautéed spinach cooked in ghee or served with slices of avocado

Lunch: Bison burger (naked) with side salad (great way to get lots of healthy plants into your diet) and some berries for dessert

Dinner: Chicken breast with broccoli and sweet potatoes

The Trio of Biotics: Probiotics, Prebiotics, and Postbiotics

Probiotics

You've probably already read about these or even taken them to improve your gut health. Probiotics are live microorganisms, typically bacteria or yeasts, that provide health benefits when consumed in adequate amounts. They are often referred to as "good" or "friendly" bacteria because they help maintain or restore a healthy balance in the gut microbiome. They are also known to improve our metabolism, support our immune system, aid in blood sugar regulation, and reduce inflammation.

Examples of probiotics: Fermented foods like yogurt, kefir, kombucha (aim for lower-sugar options), fermented veggies, miso, natto, specific types of cheese (like provolone and Parmesan, that have been aged but not heated) and apple cider vinegar. As a starting point, eat one or two servings per day.

FERMENTED FUN

How can you incorporate more fermented foods into your diet? A little goes a long way:

- Add a spoonful of sauerkraut or kimchi to tuna or salmon salad or coleslaw.
- Whisk miso into sauces and dressings (miso is salty and adds umami, so think of it for all kinds of sauces, not just Asian-inspired ones).
- Add kefir to smoothies.
- Toss a forkful of sauerkraut into your regular salad.
- Quell a craving for crunch with a pickle.
- Use the liquid from jarred fermented pickles or sauerkraut. Drink a shot after a workout (trust me on this, it's so refreshing), add a splash to dressing, or use it in a mocktail.

Prebiotics

These help facilitate the growth of probiotics—the "good" bacteria in your gut—such as bifidobacteria and lactobacilli, and in turn make them more effective. These nondigestible fibers are being studied for their potential to mitigate menopause-related health issues, including osteoporosis, periodontal disease, obesity, breast cancer, and more. By enhancing the abundance of beneficial bacteria, prebiotics may help counteract the negative effects of gut dysbiosis observed during menopause. To get more prebiotics in your system, eat yams, potatoes, and other tubers; ginger, leeks, and onions; flax and chia seeds; beans and chickpeas; fibrous fruits like berries; and vegetables.

Prebiotic fibers are resistant to digestion in the upper gastrointestinal tract, allowing them to reach the colon intact. Once in the colon, they are fermented by gut bacteria, producing short-chain fatty acids like butyrate, acetate, and propionate, which have various health benefits.

Incorporate prebiotic-rich foods into your diet daily; find three or four options that you like and alternate throughout the week.

Examples of prebiotics: Jerusalem artichokes, green bananas, onions, leeks, asparagus, garlic, apples, chicory root, dandelion greens, mushrooms, cocoa powder, flaxseed.

Postbiotics

Think of postbiotics as the baby of pre- and probiotics. Probiotic bacteria produce these compounds when they consume prebiotics (fiber). Although postbiotics have been historically considered the waste products of probiotic bacteria, we now know they offer various health benefits to your body that were once considered the effects of prebiotics and probiotics. There are a few different kinds of postbiotics, but the most important for nutritional purposes are SCFAs, which you read about earlier in this book. The study of postbiotics is relatively young, but research has shown they have properties that may help strengthen your immune system and help with nutrient absorption and energy production, and reduce inflammation.

Wondering how to get these into your diet? Because postbiotics are made from fermentation by healthy bacteria in your gut, you can naturally increase your production of them by eating prebiotic- and probiotic-rich foods.

Examples of postbiotics: Fermented foods like yogurt, sauerkraut, pickled veggies, and kombucha, which are produced by various bacterial and fungal species.

Signaling Molecules

Signaling molecules may be a new term for you, but these oh-so-important substances (specifically nitric oxide, polyphenols, and urolithin A) have a positive effect on the microbiome. I often compare the body to a busy city with many workers (your cells) bustling about and doing their work. Well, they need tools to stay healthy and keep everything running smoothly. These are signaling molecules, which give instructions that tell these workers what to do. There are many, but for the purposes of this book we are limiting it to urolithin A, nitric oxide, and polyphenols. These signaling molecules play a crucial role in promoting anti-inflammatory, antioxidant, metabolic, and longevity effects, which are particularly important during aging and menopause.

Nitric oxide (NO) is naturally produced by your body, and its most important job is getting blood, nutrients, and oxygen to travel efficiently throughout the body. It also significantly influences the gut microbiome by altering its composition and function, primarily through its antibacterial properties, impacting gut barrier integrity, and potentially impacting inflammation.

But as we age, lower estrogen means lower levels of nitric oxide, as estrogen is a trigger for NO production. Such low levels have been shown to play a role in cardiovascular disease, and because NO has an important role in oxygen delivery to the cells, promoting cellular renewal and vitality, its decline will affect how we age throughout the body. The higher levels of nitric oxide normally seen in premenopausal women provide cardioprotective effects and inhibit the propagation of smooth muscle typically seen in heart disease. So, with the transition into menopause, our lower levels of estrogen lead to lower levels of nitric oxide and the loss of this very important protection inside our blood vessels.

Foods high in nitrates: Nitrates are found in nuts and green vegetables like celery, arugula, spinach, broccoli, cabbage, parsley, and fennel, as well as root veggies like beets, carrots, and radishes, and pumpkin. You can also take nitric oxide supplements, but quality is key! And stay away from nitrate-*added* foods like processed meats and bacon.

Polyphenols: These are the favorite food sources of our gut microbiome. The GM metabolizes them into smaller, more easily absorbed molecules and makes them more bioactive. They nourish your beneficial gut bacteria, fostering a robust environment that helps them outnumber harmful bacteria. Eating a polyphenol-rich diet can enhance the production of other signaling molecules (specifically urolithin A and resveratrol), supporting overall health.

Polyphenols may act in the gut microbiota to favor the increase of beneficial bacteria and hamper the increase of pathogenic bacteria. They can also potentially lower blood sugar, reduce inflammation, and lower blood pressure—but everyone is different. Polyphenol metabolism is very bio-individual; research suggests that some people absorb more or less depending on the health of their microbiome. This is where supplementation can be vital.

Foods high in polyphenols: Vibrant foods like leafy greens, cruciferous vegetables, green tea, certain spices, high-quality olive oil, and even dark chocolate.

GO GREEN (TEA)

You can use green tea in other ways besides drinking it. Poach chicken or fish in it, or poach fruit in it for a healthy dessert. Add it to smoothies. Mix it with broth as a base for soup.

Urolithin A, a naturally occurring compound derived from the metabolism of gut microbiota, does double duty as a postbiotic and a signaling molecule. It is derived from ellagic acid, which is found in many foods, including berries, pomegranates, nuts, and spices. The gut microbiota breaks down these foods and releases it as a postbiotic. Urolithin A has the potential to enhance muscle health and performance by improving mitochondrial function and regulating autophagy during fasting, but it can also be activated with certain types of exercise and heat or cold exposure.

Like other polyphenolic compounds, urolithin A absorption is highly bio-individual; only about 30 percent of the population has the right mix of bacteria in their gut to produce urolithin A from polyphenols. This is yet another reason why maintaining a healthy gut microbiome in menopause is so important; we need it optimized to create these kinds of compounds to support our health.

Foods that stimulate urolithin A: Fruits like pomegranates, raspberries, and strawberries, and nuts like walnuts and almonds.

Water, Water, Water

I can't say it more bluntly than this: Hydration is critically important for all women, and especially as we get older, we begin to see a higher risk for dehydration. During menopause, thirst mechanisms can become less sensitive due to hormonal changes, particularly with the decline in estrogen (there it is again!), as it plays a role in regulating fluid balance and how the brain senses thirst. Estrogen also boosts osmotic sensitivity, helping the body to retain water. As estrogen and progesterone decrease during menopause, so does this fluid-retention ability. This does not mean fluid retention in a negative sense, simply that our loss of estrogen impacts our ability to hold on to water and stay hydrated. When estrogen and progesterone drop, some women may experience decreased thirst perception, leading to a higher risk of dehydration.

Suggested water intake: half your body weight. If you are 150 pounds, try to get 75 ounces a day. I make sure I get my minimum by filling a 60-ounce glass pitcher every morning, so that I have a visual reminder of how much water I need to consume each day. I will also add in electrolytes, and I'll drink herbal teas or green tea depending on my mood.

What to Avoid

These are typically food groups I have my patients steer clear of when they are trying to maximize their nutritional plan.

Gluten: I am sure you have heard a lot about the debate about gluten. A protein found in wheat, barley, and rye, gluten has changed a great deal since our ancestors first started consuming it; the modern-day version is highly inflammatory. In 2000, scientists at the University of Maryland discovered the existence of a protein called zonulin, which is produced by our bodies whenever we eat gluten. Zonulin opens the tight junctions in our small intestine's lining—yep, leaky gut. This is super important because 60 percent of our immune system is right under this one-cell layer of our small intestine.

Given we've seen a 400 percent rise in the number of Americans with celiac (an autoimmune disorder) and many of us are afflicted with NCGS (non-celiac gluten sensitivity), I generally recommend eliminating it entirely or limiting it to an occasional indulgence. There are so many gluten-free alternatives now, although these should be a temporary indulgence and not something to consume on a daily basis.

Processed sugars: Unfortunately, sugar is ubiquitous in our current nutritional paradigm. It is in everything—frozen foods, condiments, pasta sauce, bread, just to name a few—and our taste buds are wildly attuned to it. Unlike glucose, which can be used by nearly every cell in the body, fructose is processed almost exclusively by our liver. When we consume processed table sugar (sucrose), our body breaks it down into glucose and fructose and sends the fructose straight to our liver, where through a process called lipogenesis, it is converted into fats such as triglycerides and cholesterol. Even worse is HFCS (high-fructose corn syrup), which is cheap, and the processed-food industry uses it with vigor.

Fructose drives much of the metabolic disease we see today, including heart disease, diabetes, fatty liver, cancer, depression, premature aging of our skin, weight gain, and poor metabolic health . . . just for starters. If you need to sweeten something, use fruit, raw honey, coconut sugar, maple syrup, or stevia leaf.

DAIRY: GOOD OR BAD?

Dairy is a conundrum. In my practice I have found that most middle-aged women have some degree of dairy sensitivity. Many are also lactose intolerant. Don't buy into the hype that we need dairy to protect our bones; we can get lots of calcium from other dietary sources, like sesame seeds, sardines, collard greens, spinach, salmon, and more.

If you tolerate dairy, stick to organic full-fat yogurt, kefir, grass-fed butter, ghee, or even cheese. I find that many of my patients do best with either A2 (less inflammatory) cow milk products or sheep or goat's milk, as they are more easily digestible. Grass-fed options are even better, as they have a superior omega-3-to-omega-6 ratio (optimal is 1:1). Raw milk remains controversial; the federal government made it a crime to sell unpasteurized dairy across state lines in 2016, and twenty states have outlawed all sales of raw milk.

Seed oils: The average American consumes five to ten tablespoons of seed or vegetable oil per day, usually unknowingly. These include canola, corn, cottonseed, grape-seed, rice bran, safflower, sunflower, and soybean oils. Soybean oil, in particular, is the most consumed oil in the US. A study at University of California, Riverside, showed in animal models that soybean oil not only leads to obesity and diabetes but could also affect neurological conditions like autism, Alzheimer's disease, anxiety, and depression. All of these oils are high in unstable omega-6 fatty acids that can break down into toxins when you cook them.

In ancient times, humans obtained "pro-inflammatory" omega-6 and "anti-inflammatory" omega-3 fatty acids in a certain ratio that has been estimated to be 1:1. However, in the past century or so, this ratio has shifted dramatically due to the Standard American Diet and may now be as high as 20:1 omega-6 to omega-3. Too much omega-6 to omega 3 contributes to chronic inflammation, which damages the lining of blood vessels and the membranes of our cells and generates a huge amount of free radicals that damage cells further.

There are other issues with seed oils: With excessive consumption, they disrupt our metabolism and create metabolic disease, like diabetes. At a certain concentration, these fatty acids shut down the ability of our mitochondria to generate energy. To survive, they're forced to draw more sugar from the bloodstream, which depletes our blood glucose. When our blood sugar drops (reactive hypoglycemia), it generates powerful sugar cravings. So, a diet high in seed oils can actually contribute to carb cravings and a desire for sugar. Eek. Read your labels and ask what they use in your favorite restaurants to prepare your meals—don't be afraid to be your own advocate.

Alcohol: At this point in my adult life, I don't find alcohol to be a worthy part of my lifestyle. I used to enjoy an occasional extra-dirty martini, but as I headed into perimenopause, I found that alcohol was way too disruptive to my sleep and even one martini gave me a horrific hangover the following day, not to mention hot flashes, which further disrupted my very precious sleep. Alcohol exacerbates hot flashes; the research demonstrates that the women with the worst hot flashes typically are the least healthy, although the cause and effect between alcohol use and hot flashes is unknown.

Let's talk about why alcohol may not benefit your health in middle age and beyond:

- It damages the microbiome, can lead to histamine response, and promotes leaky gut and endotoxemia (a condition in which endotoxins like lipopolysaccharides [LPS] enter the bloodstream, often due to a leaky gut).
- It stimulates us to eat nutrient-devoid foods and stimulates our appetites, which can lead to overeating.

- It makes it harder to maintain healthy muscle and bones. These two areas are critically important as we get older; we want to avoid developing sarcopenia and osteoporosis.
- It is terrible for sleep, as it reduces REM sleep, blunts melatonin secretion, and can make us more prone to vasomotor symptoms and hot flashes.
- It's terrible for our brains and shrinks our hippocampus, which is the commander of our stress-response system (HPA axis).
- It impairs the metabolism of estrogen, which can impact our risk for breast cancer. One drink per day increases our risk by 7 to 10 percent.

So, what does this all mean? I generally suggest eliminating or limiting alcohol; enjoy it at special celebrations, such as weddings or birthdays, but don't make it part of your day-to-day lifestyle if you are concerned about any of the research I have discussed.

What Else to Avoid

Antibiotics: When used appropriately and sparingly, antibiotics can be a literal lifesaver, as they help fight potentially deadly infections. But today, they are often overused and overprescribed. Check out these statistics:

- In 2022, 236.4 million antibiotic prescriptions were dispensed from US community pharmacies, roughly 7 prescriptions for every 10 people in the outpatient setting.
- At least 28 percent of antibiotic prescriptions are written unnecessarily in US doctor's offices and emergency departments.
- In 2020, the United States sold 13.23 million pounds of "medically important" antibiotics for use in farm animals. This is used to prevent infections but also as a way to fatten livestock and poultry faster prior to slaughter. Ingesting antibiotics this way will only mess up our own microbiome.

Antibiotic use can have several negative effects on the gut microbiota, including reduced species diversity, altered metabolic activity, and the selection of antibiotic-resistant organisms, which in turn can lead to antibiotic-associated diarrhea and recurrent *Clostridioides difficile* infections. I have seen far too many patients develop long-term issues from improperly prescribed antibiotics, including leaky gut, susceptibility to autoimmune disorders, and more. Until there is greater care in prescription rates, be diligent about what you put in your body.

THE ABCs OF EDCs

Toxins are all around us. Whether it's pollutants in the air, chemicals in our hygiene products, or pesticides on our food, we need to be careful about what we expose ourselves to for our health, and we are learning that we must be even more vigilant in middle age. A cumulative exposure to endocrine-disrupting chemicals (EDCs) throughout our lifetime via personal-care products, food, and environment can worsen symptoms of the perimenopause transition, and recent evidence suggests that exposure to EDCs may cause early onset of menopause. While that sounds scary, there are plenty of easy things we can do to mitigate these harmful substances.

First things first: What are EDCs? These natural or man-made chemicals present in all sorts of products are typically used to protect them—such as keeping food safe from pests, extending the shelf life of your favorite foundation, or making your rug stain-resistant. Unfortunately, we have found out that what makes the products good can be bad for us. Many of these chemicals have been shown to alter our hormones and have been linked to a variety of other health problems, such as metabolic disorders, increased cancer risk, leaky gut, and immune suppression. Yet these harmful chemicals are still being used widely. What can we do about it? First is to know thy enemy. Here is a list of the major chemicals to stay away from:

Bisphenol A (BPA) is often found in polycarbonate plastics, such as water bottles, baby bottles, and food packaging, including the lining in cans—even paper receipts. Note: Organic canned foods can still have an epoxy plastic BPA lining.

Glyphosate is an herbicide and pesticide widely sprayed on crops and plants (infamously used in the weed killer Roundup). While the EPA hasn't recognized glyphosate as toxic, the International Agency for Research on Cancer (IARC), a part of the World Health Organization (WHO), classified glyphosate as a "probable human carcinogen" in 2015.

Per- and polyfluoroalkyl substances (PFAS) have been used for their water-, grease-, and heat-resistant properties, so these can be found in carpet, pots and pans, clothing, cosmetics, and other plastics. People can also be exposed through contaminated air, soil, and drinking water. PFAS are typically known as forever chemicals, as they are incredibly difficult to break down.

Phthalates are used to make products more flexible and durable, and are found in personal-care items such as fragrances, shampoos, creams, deodorants, and cosmetics.

Second, try to avoid EDCs at all cost. Here's a good starting point:

1. **Read labels.** Check all food, personal-care, cosmetic, and household products. Use "green" cleaners that are labeled "phosphate-free." For food, check for USDA organic, non-GMO, non-antibiotic, and hormone-free foods. As for fish, bypass the "farm-raised" fish (you never know what they have been fed) and go for wild-caught. There is a lot of greenwashing in the industry—don't be fooled by it.
2. **Filter your water.** Good water filters can remove a broad range of EDCs and other toxins—and they can make water taste better, too. If you think bottled water is better than tap water, think again: The Environmental Working Group (EWG) tested ten bestselling brands of bottled water and found thirty-eight contaminants,

including bacteria, fertilizer, and industrial chemicals, all at levels similar to those found in tap water.

3. **Be careful with cookware and storage.** Minimize plastic use wherever you can. Use glass containers and buy fewer canned goods. Avoid nonstick cookware.
4. **Regularly dust and vacuum with a HEPA filter.** This can eliminate or minimize chemicals in the air and dust. And a good air filter will help as well.
5. **Avoid the Dirty Dozen.** Each year, the EWG creates a list of foods that have the highest pesticide residues when grown conventionally (not organically). Typically, this list includes strawberries, spinach, kale, collard and mustard greens, grapes, peaches, pears, nectarines, apples, bell and hot peppers, cherries, and blueberries.

While it may seem like an overwhelming task at first, making these small changes can have a huge impact on our hormones and overall health. Your hormones will thank you for it.

Managing Weight

Remember Jennifer? After we did a full workup on her, she started the following plan:

1. She increased her hydration (half her body weight in ounces daily).
2. She slowly transitioned off most of the processed foods while tracking her macros and increasing her protein intake, aiming for thirty grams per meal. She also added some brightly colored vegetables to her diet, especially cruciferous veggies like broccoli, cauliflower, and arugula.

3. She started tracking her step count and working with a personal trainer to help her safely begin integrating more physical activity, including body-weight exercises. (We'll talk more about the importance of exercise in the next chapter.)
4. She got more sleep; she was previously getting only five to six hours a night, and we were able to convince her to increase her sleep to seven hours a night and get off electronics prior to bedtime.

Within six weeks, we did a Zoom call, and I could see the difference in her energy, coloring, and mood immediately. She told me that she was having at least one good poop daily and she felt less bloated; she had lost two inches from her waist, and her clothes fit so much better. Once she realized that eating more protein was so satiating and that her cravings were greatly diminished, we started to add back in more carbs, such as non-starchy veggies, low-glycemic berries, and a small serving of fermented veggies daily. Small wins go a long way. I've learned to keep my clients' plans simple and structured. It can be overwhelming to make too many changes all at once, so it helps to introduce them gradually. I always say small steps eventually lead to big gains.

Putting It All Together

What should your nutritional plan for middlepause health look like? Are you struggling with a lack of energy? Weight gain? Joint pain? Bloating? I don't love the concept of diets in general, as most are overly restrictive and limiting, and let's face it, they are typically a temporary solution to a long-term problem. Often the key to weight loss is simple: adherence to whole foods, irrespective of the particular macronutrient composition, rather than processed foods. Some women do well on low-carb diets or even ketogenic diets, but the success can often be attributable to the specific composition of the gut microbiome in each individual. In other words, if someone has been consuming ultraprocessed foods and is not metabolically healthy, their gut microbiome will be different than that of someone who is on a healthier diet. Similarly, lowered estrogen states, like in late perimenopause and menopause, may make it harder to break down and emulsify fats—so if someone goes keto or low carb and experiences weight gain, gas, bloating, and brain fog, it may be a sign that it is the wrong diet for them.

That's why I recommend following an anti-inflammatory diet. This is about consuming foods that are less likely to drive inflammation in the body. The biggest offenders that are often cut from the diet are: gluten, grains, dairy, sugar, and alcohol. Sometimes, just removing these foods can make a huge impact on energy and alleviate any symptoms someone may have with a specific food. Beyond this, it is the magic of focusing on the highest-quality nutrients your budget permits. That means thirty grams of protein per meal and brightly pigmented fruits and vegetables. Aim for two or three vegetables and one piece of fruit per day. Layer in healthy fats. Keeping it simple equates with sustainability.

I try to find sustainable solutions for my clients. What works for one woman may not work for another, and while we always start with a less processed diet, we experiment with macros and meal frequency to find what works for each.

When to Eat Is Just as Important as What to Eat

There has been some amazing research that shows if we time our meals in specific ways, we can reap great benefits from it. There is great value in digestive rest—a gentler form of popularized intermittent fasting that can help support the microbiome without too much stress on the body. What do I mean by digestive rest? It's about twelve to thirteen hours of not eating, giving your body a break from processing food. Intermittent fasting has a longer window of not eating—sixteen hours—and eating within an eight-hour time period. Research suggests a strong connection between the gut microbiome, middlepause, and fasting, indicating that fasting may influence the microbiome composition and help regulate changes in the gut bacteria composition during menopause that can impact metabolic health, potentially alleviating some menopausal symptoms; however, more research is needed to fully understand the mechanisms involved.

It has been my clinical experience that many women begin with IF and slowly start eating less and less food . . . until they get to a point where they are so calorically restricted that we have to back off. I'm a huge believer in the value of IF, but only with the understanding that we are supposed to be nurturing our bodies and not living in a state of chronic deprivation. So, I prefer to suggest twelve hours of digestive rest as a means to (a) keep eating and not eating in specific time frames, and (b) permit my patients to consume two to three meals per day with a minimum of one hundred grams of protein per day and ensure that they are meeting their protein needs.

Once your nutrition goals are in a good place, the next step is to match them with an exercise plan that works for you. Let's talk about how we can move our bodies to best maximize our health in middlepause.

Chapter Summary

1. Aim for thirty to fifty grams of protein at every meal.
2. Track your macros to see where your needs are.
3. Aim for thirty grams of unprocessed carbs per meal and add in healthy fats as needed.
4. Be conscientious about reading labels; knowledge is power! Don't hesitate to ask how your food is being prepared at restaurants.
5. Hydrate!

References for this chapter can be found on my website: cynthiathurlow.com/themenopausegut-references

Chapter 7

Keep Moving

When I was in my thirties and early forties, I did intense classes at our local gym. I was a huge fan of their hardcore conditioning classes and was waking up at *four a.m.* to take five a.m. classes, shower, and then head to the hospital. I did this for years. When I got to age forty-four, I started to think, *I'm not recovering like I used to.* I also noticed my periods were insanely heavy, and I was just so tired all the time. W*hat am I doing to myself? Am I forcing myself to do something that may no longer be in my best interest? Is all this intensity good for my middle-aged body?*

It was a reframing that I needed to think about, and also one I ask you to think about. This stage of our life is an opportunity to change not just our mindset, but also the way we treat ourselves. Changes in our hormones impact our body composition. We are more prone to inflammation in the setting of low estrogen, progesterone, and, in most instances, testosterone.

No matter how athletic you have been, changes in middlepause are going to make you see that we can't keep the same pace as we did when we were eighteen. Just like nutrition, exercise can offset your natural aging and menopausal changes. The best types of exercise for aging bodies are those that build muscle, get our heart pumping a bit, and help support our bones.

Reasons to "Just Do It"

More than forty-seven million women worldwide enter the menopause transition every year. More than 70 percent of them will experience musculoskeletal symptoms, and 25 percent will be so affected that it will be disabling. This often unrecognized condition is largely influenced by estrogen changes and includes joint pain, inflammation, loss of muscle mass, and loss of bone density, which leads to an increased risk of frailty, falls, and osteoarthritis—in other words, the condition called MSSM, as we discussed in chapter 5. Do you know what will help prevent much of this downward spiral? Exercise.

How beneficial can exercise be for menopause?

- Exercise improves our overall well-being by combating the negative effects of declining estrogen levels on the body, which will help manage a plethora of menopause symptoms like hot flashes.
- It can help create a calorie deficit and minimize midlife weight gain.
- It increases bone mass. Strength training and impact activities (like walking or running) can help to offset the decline of bone mineral density and prevent osteoporosis.
- It reduces low back pain.
- It is proven to help reduce stress and improve mood.
- It can lower the risk of dementia and improve the cognitive function of middle-aged women.
- Increasing muscle mass and function can help prevent and alleviate sarcopenia.
- It increases our balance, flexibility, and overall physical function.
- It reduces the risk of cardiovascular disease in postmenopausal women.
- Both aerobic exercise and strength exercises can counteract the changes associated with poor metabolic health in sedentary menopausal women.

Exercise Works Out the Gut

If those benefits aren't enough to convince you to pull out your trainers, maybe knowing that exercise can help restore your gut will help. Exercise has been shown to positively influence the microbiome, mitigating some of the negative effects of menopause on gut health, although further studies are needed to fully understand the complex interactions between these factors. Research suggests that more physical activity, measured in METs (metabolic equivalents, or how much energy your body uses during physical activity compared with when at rest), had the greatest predictive value of diversity in the microbiome. Also, exercise may increase the abundance of certain types of bacteria associated with anti-inflammation, such as verrucomicrobia, which can reduce the abundance of bacteria associated with pro-inflammation.

While single bouts of high-volume exercise can influence the gut microbiota, there is research showing how consistency is key: Moderate- to high-intensity intervals for thirty to ninety minutes at least three times a week for at least eight weeks have been shown to provide the most consistent improvements to the gut microbiota.

Let's see all this data work in real time. I worked with a fifty-year-old client named Darby. She was perimenopausal, with a BMI of 32 and a strong desire to lose weight. And she had good reason to lose it: She had chronic knee pain. Osteoarthritis showed up on her X-ray, and it didn't help that she was carrying around extra weight that added to that pain. Being just ten pounds overweight puts an extra fifteen to fifty pounds of pressure on your knees.

Even worse, her job as an administrative assistant at a car dealership was sedentary but high-stress. She didn't prioritize exercise. She wasn't able to eat when she was hungry, so she binged in the evening. Being overweight and inactive exacerbated her inflammation, it was a never ending cycle.

"And it's not just my knee, Cynthia. I feel stiff in my hips, ankles, even my wrists! I am fifty, not eighty!" she cried. "I notice more body fat in areas that I didn't have it before, and I feel like I am losing muscle definition."

I did a workup on her, and her labs were consistent with patterns for borderline diabetes and high blood pressure, and they showed signs of osteopenia, which she'd never heard of.

"Osteopenia what?" she asked. Like so many other women, she had not been counseled on the changes that occur with the middlepause transition that can not only impact bone but also lead to musculoskeletal syndrome of menopause.

I suggested a two-part plan for her: (1) an anti-inflammatory diet that would eliminate gluten, grains, processed sugars, and alcohol, with thirty to fifty grams of protein per meal, along with a supplement regimen of creatine monohydrate and vitamin D_3 with K_2; and (2) an exercise routine with an experienced personal trainer, who started her with body-weight exercises, which later progressed to weight training with higher weight and lower reps, which, as we explain later in this chapter, research shows is best for middle-aged women.

Within six weeks, she had lost *twenty* pounds and had less joint pain. She also felt that she had fewer food cravings, and she was more motivated to exercise, so we added in walking at lunchtime for fifteen to twenty minutes, increasing her daily steps to five thousand. Her blood sugar levels, while not great, were definitely going in the right direction. She used a glucometer to check her blood sugar several times a day. The best outcome was that she continued with this program and really started to feel and look better.

Maybe you aren't the same as Darby—maybe you regularly work out already, or feel like you have a good diet plan. Everyone is different—someone might be a lifelong distance runner racking up their bib numbers, a dancer, or someone who barely made it to the gym to make their membership worthwhile. No matter where your baseline physical fitness is, bio-individuality rules, and you have to see what works for you. That said, there are two core pieces that I did with Darby that will work for anyone in menopause: Move, and eat for your gut.

Whatever You Do, Just Move

At this stage of our lives, it's not about topping a mileage or beating a personal best. The focus here is on musculoskeletal health and strength to counteract hormonal decline. Remember that loss of muscle begets loss of strength, which then leads to frailty and falls. We want to focus on being strong more than being thin. For all of us who grew weight-obsessed and fat-phobic in the 1980s and '90s, this mindset shift may take some effort!

Type I muscle fibers are slow-twitch fibers and are designed to help with endurance work, whereas type II muscle fibers are designed for power. As we age, we see a faster decline in type II fibers, which can result in sarcopenia, reduced strength, and slower reaction times.

The loss of type II muscle fibers, specifically, is what leads to changes in how we live our lives, so we want to remain strong and independent as long as possible.

Did you know that declining estrogen is associated with the loss of type II muscle fibers (and subsequently their power), which has been suggested as the primary measure for completing everyday activities? We're talking basics here, such as bathing, dressing, and eating. Additionally, the loss of muscle cells leads to increased inflammation and decreased muscle mass and strength—that is, sarcopenia. Physical inactivity not only places women's health at risk, it also increases menopausal problems. So, the emerging answer is that exercise just might be the most promising nonpharmaceutical intervention.

What kind, exactly? Studies suggest that a mix of strength training and high-intensity exercise will give you the best bang for your buck. One study showed that HIIT (high-intensity interval training) and resistance training are effective in reducing that unwanted abdominal/visceral fat, as well as improving intestinal microbiota composition and insulin sensitivity. There isn't any set recommendation for how much you should do, but there are guidelines for what will benefit you. And remember, while you can't target visceral fat with a bunch of crunches, exercise should help with metabolic changes and with hormone-driven body composition changes overall.

Strength First

Many women don't prioritize resistance training, but it becomes critically important as we age. There are many variables that determine what types of exercise are more beneficial, but based on my clinical experience and the available research, strength training is crucial for maintaining muscle mass and building muscle and strength. We know that we lose 10 percent of our bone mass in the first five years of menopause, and that's when we're at greatest risk for osteoporosis. When someone was diagnosed with osteoporosis twenty years ago, that was it—you might as well cover yourself with Bubble Wrap.

Strength training during menopause will offset the bone loss that happens as a result of hormone changes, and it offers numerous health benefits, including improved muscle mass, bone density, and reduction of menopausal symptoms such as hot flashes. One study implemented a fifteen-week resistance-training program in which menopausal women performed specific exercises three times per week. Each session included eight exercises, executed in two sets of eight to twelve repetitions. This regimen led to a significant decrease in the frequency of moderate to severe hot flashes. Another meta-analysis reviewed multiple randomized controlled trials and found that resistance-training programs, typically conducted two to three times per week, improved muscle strength, bone density, and overall quality of life in menopausal women. This same study shows how strength exercises can improve menopausal symptoms that affect muscle performance such as heart rate and hot flashes.

So, it is safe to say, then, that menopausal women should engage in strength-training exercises two to three times per week. Each session should involve multiple exercises focusing on major muscle groups, with two to three sets of eight to twelve repetitions per exercise, and then you can increase your weights and lower your reps as you progress. Start with manageable weights and gradually increase intensity under professional guidance to ensure safety and effectiveness.

How much weight is right? Everybody's interpretation of *heavy* is different, but we want to be lifting heavy-enough weights that we trigger the changes we need, but not so much that we hurt ourselves.

If you are new to exercise or are inexperienced with weight training, I highly suggest working with an experienced personal trainer who understands how to guide middle-aged women properly. There are also lots of resources online that include videos and additional materials to help guide and support you in these endeavors.

If you have a cardiologist, pulmonologist, or other specialist, make sure that they are aware of your desire to become more physically active. They may have recommendations or suggestions for how best to proceed as well.

Here are some suggested guidelines for getting started with training—and remember, safety first!

1. **Start with 2 or 3 Days Per Week**
    - Begin with 2 or 3 strength-training sessions per week (on nonconsecutive days).
    - Sessions should last 30 to 45 minutes, including warm-up and cooldown.
2. **Focus on Major Muscle Groups**

    Each session should target all major muscle groups:
    - **Legs** (squats, lunges)
    - **Back** (rows, lat pulldowns)
    - **Chest** (push-ups, bench press)
    - **Arms** (biceps curls, triceps dips)
    - **Core** (planks, dead bugs)
3. **Use Light Weights and Perfect Form**
    - Begin with light weights or resistance bands to learn proper form.
    - Aim for 2 or 3 sets of 8 to 12 reps per exercise.
    - Slow and controlled movements reduce injury risk.
    - Increase weight gradually as you build strength.

The goal is to work your way up to heavier weights that necessitate only doing four to six reps; this is what stimulates muscle best, according to Dr. Vonda Wright, orthopedic surgeon and expert in musculoskeletal aging.

4. Prioritize Bone Health and Joint Safety

- Menopause increases the risk of osteoporosis, so focus on weight-bearing and resistance exercises.
- Avoid excessive high-impact movements if you have joint pain.
- Strengthen stabilizing muscles (hips, knees, core) to prevent falls.

5. Incorporate Functional and Balance Exercises

- Balance training (e.g., single-leg stands, yoga) reduces fall risk.
- Functional movements (e.g., squats, step-ups) mimic daily activities, improving mobility.

6. Warm-up and Cooldown Are Essential

- Warm-up (5–10 min.): Light cardio + dynamic stretching (arm circles, leg swings)
- Cooldown (5 min.): Static stretching + deep breathing to reduce muscle soreness

7. Prioritize Recovery and Nutrition

- Rest days are crucial for muscle repair—avoid training the same muscles two days in a row.
- Eat adequate protein, with a minimum of a hundred grams per day to support muscle growth.
- Stay hydrated and fuel up with whole foods (lean proteins, healthy fats, complex carbs).

8. Listen to Your Body and Modify When Needed

- If an exercise causes pain, modify it or try an alternative.
- If experiencing hot flashes, exercise in a cooler environment or choose morning or evening sessions, and discuss with your healthcare provider whether you need adjustments in your HRT.

9. Combine with Other Exercises for Best Results

- Cardiovascular zone 2 training (e.g., low- to moderate-intensity walking, swimming, cycling): 30 to 40 minutes 2 or 3 days per week
- Flexibility and mobility work (yoga, Pilates) to help prevent stiffness

10. **Be Patient and Stay Consistent**
    - Progress takes time, but strength training reduces menopausal symptoms, boosts mood, and improves overall well-being. Keep a positive mindset, track progress, and celebrate small victories! As I tell my patients and clients, you cannot track what you do not measure.

Pump It Up

What form of exercise is best for our health, particularly gut health? Research has shown that few to no changes in the gut microbiota were seen with resistance training alone, and most changes in the gut are more likely to be caused by aerobic exercise. Get this: One incredible study found that aerobic exercise changed the microbiota within two weeks of beginning exercise and established a stable new composition between six and eight weeks. Crazy, right?

What makes exercise aerobic, exactly? This involves cardiovascular work that elevates your heart rate and increases your intake of oxygen. In other words, movement that gets you huffing and puffing—in a good way. The latest science points to what we call getting in the zone—zone 2, to be exact. Zoned training uses our heart rate as a guide for effort. Zone 5 is your VO_2 max, with zone 2 at 60 to 70 percent of your maximum heart rate. Zone 2 is also known as the fat-burning zone. For the average person, that's heart rate of 120 to 130. For those who have osteoporosis, you are not off the hook. If running is not in the cards, you can jump rope or rebound on a trampoline. (That's what NASA astronauts do when they come back from a mission, often with a bone deficit.)

Lastly, you want to be consistent—think the long game, as exercise programs lasting more than thirty days provide even more beneficial changes. Remember that finding the right combination of exercises for you and your lifestyle is key. Be open-minded to trying new forms of exercise and ensure you are getting adequate recovery in between.

It's All About Balance

Remember the fairy tale about Goldilocks? The principle works here, too: You don't want to do too much exercise or too little. Research suggests that the right amount of exercise is crucial, along with the intensity. As we navigate middlepause, we want to be mindful of how much hormetic stress we are placing on our bodies. Intensity of exercise is a double-edged sword because anything *too* high-intensity, especially for a long time, can be harmful to our health. To find a balance, I suggest starting with two or three days a week to kick-start the benefits to the microbiome, progressing to five days a week to really maximize those benefits. Anything more and you might put yourself at risk for overexercising. And this can compromise gut-barrier function and potentially create a leaky gut. Pushing yourself too hard, for too long, or at the wrong times (like when you have had a terrible night's sleep or are immune-compromised, jet-lagged, etc.) can be too stressful on the body and potentially increase cortisol to unwanted levels, leaving you feeling quite depleted. You'll know you've pushed too much if after an intense workout you needed to take a nap, or if you find yourself getting sick more frequently or you have an increase in overall body or muscle soreness.

A Sample Training Program

I suggest the following as a starter kit that includes aerobic exercise and resistance training; it should aim for two hours and thirty minutes of zone 2 activity each week. Be aware of your target heart rate range and track the intensity of exercise by employing the talk test (you should be able to talk without too much effort). You can supplement this with deep breathing, yoga, and stretching exercises, which will help to manage the stress of life and menopause-related symptoms.

Ideal exercise plan:

1. Weight training: 2 or 3 sessions per week
2. Zone 2 workout: 2 or 3 sessions per week. Walking is fine, just track your steps, aiming for a minimum of 5,000 per day.
3. HIIT: 1 or 2 sessions a week. Example: Sprint for 20 to 30 seconds, followed by 2 minutes of walking. Do this for 3 or 4 rounds (this is short in duration).
4. Incorporate flexibility work as you can (gentle yoga, Pilates, or stretching).

Do what you can—and always try to improve. Dr. Stacy Sims, a researcher and exercise physiologist, recommends lifting heavy weights with fewer reps to help muscles grow and communicate with nerves. She also suggests incorporating plyometrics, high-intensity endurance training, and adaptogenic supplements (more on them in chapter 12) into your routine.

What If You Haven't Been Physically Active for a Long Time?

This a step-by-step guide to get you off the couch and exercising if you have let your gym membership lapse . . . years ago.

1. If you are new to exercise, please find a personal trainer, in-person or online, who is experienced with working with middle-aged clients. This can help you learn proper technique and not injure yourself in the process.
2. Do a baseline assessment: Use a bioimpedance/body composition scale or get a DXA scan (which helps to measure fat-free mass to lean body mass), or, if you are unable to get access to these, you can use a measuring tape to get a baseline assessment of your waist-to-hip ratio (WHR). This measurement can help assess your risk for

certain health conditions. Divide your waist circumference by your hip circumference. A ratio greater than 0.8 for women or 0.94 for men increases your risk of metabolic complications. A WHR of 1.0 or higher is often considered high-risk for heart disease and other health problems.

3. Waist circumference: A simple tape measure can help you track your waistline. Measure your waist at your belly button. A waist circumference greater than 35 inches for women is a component of poor metabolic health and warrants further evaluation.
4. If you have chronic health issues, you may need to get a medical evaluation before starting any exercise program, especially if you have chronic cardiac, respiratory, or renal health issues. When in doubt, let your healthcare team know that you are interested in becoming more physically active.
5. Start with walking after meals for 10 to 15 minutes.
6. Incorporate stretching into your routine. Start with 5 minutes a day and build from there.
7. Start with body-weight exercises (personal trainer or online resources). Ideally, 2 or 3 days per week for at least 30 minutes, working diligently at progressive overload, which means increasing weight or intensity over time.
8. Foster better flexibility by trying muscle-stretching workouts, such as yoga, Pilates, or tai chi. Aim for 1 or 2 times a week.
9. Integrate zone 2 training into your lifestyle.
10. Gradually add in some HIIT, 1 or 2 times a week.
11. Incorporate some type of cooldown into your workout.

Always ensure you are getting enough quality sleep to help support recovery from physical activity.

More advanced:

1. Aim for 5,000 to 10,000 steps per day, which you can track with your smartphone, Apple Watch, or a fitness tracker, like a Whoop band.
2. While still weight training (progressive overload) 2 or 3 days per week, add HIIT, as described on page 137.
3. Wear a weighted vest or weight belt (see page 141) to add a bit of resistance to the workouts and add axial skeletal muscle load. Your axial skeleton is composed of your skull, spine, and rib cage, eighty bones in total!

Flexibility Is Important, Too

Flexibility is important as we get older—we want to be limber and strong so we can exercise every day. Stretching is great; doing it daily for ten to fifteen minutes suppresses our sympathetic nervous system activity and increases vagal tone and parasympathetic activity, reducing stress in the body. It also has a positive impact on psychological well-being and can improve sleep quality.

Gentle stretching practices like yoga improve our vagal tone (the activity of the vagus nerve, which is the main nerve in the parasympathetic nervous system), decrease our heart rate and blood pressure, decrease pain, and optimize immune function. Additionally, it's been associated with improved vitality, reduction in anger, anxiety, tension, depression, and fatigue, as well as improved quality of life. (Those ancient yogis were onto something, weren't they?)

Figuring Out Your Zone 2

Engaging in zone 2 activities, such as low- to moderate-level walking, cycling, or swimming, for at least thirty minutes on most days can improve cardiovascular fitness, aid in weight management, and improve metabolic health. Additionally, this training intensity helps regulate cortisol levels, reducing stress and its associated impacts during menopause.

How to calculate your zone 2 exercise: Remember, your heart rate should be 60 to 70 percent of your maximum heart rate. To estimate your max heart rate, multiply your age by 0.7, then subtract that number from 208. Then, take 60 and 70 percent of that number to determine your zone 2 heart-rate range. That will give you your lower threshold: 0.6 × (208 – age × 0.7). And your upper threshold: 0.7 × (208 – age × 0.7).

Incorporating zone 2 training into your routine is a valuable strategy for maintaining health and well-being during menopause.

Don't Overdo It or Hurt Yourself

Whatever you decide to do as a form of exercise, know that changes in estrogen can reduce collagen and elastin in our connective tissues, which impacts muscles, tendons, and ligaments, which then has the potential to impact joint stability and cause injury. And so, one of the common questions is: What can I do proactively to lessen the likelihood of hurting myself?

The Goldilocks effect works in the world of exercise, too—we don't want to do too little, and we don't want to overexert ourselves. Too intense exercise overtaxes the delicate HPA axis, raises cortisol, and contributes to challenges with recovery, sleep, and more, as well as increases the risk of injury. High cortisol also degrades our muscles, lowers immunity, and makes it harder to recover; the lower estrogen levels of late perimenopause and menopause make it easier to get injured, too.

- If you are still having a menstrual cycle, you can exercise harder in the follicular phase (when estrogen predominates) and need to back off in intensity during the luteal phase (when progesterone predominates).
  - Follicular phase: HIIT, personal bests, sprinting
  - Luteal phase: yoga, tai chi, body-weight exercise

- If you are not sleeping or managing your stress well, increase your physical activity, as it is known to help with sleep.

WEIGHTED VESTS, YES OR NO?

Weighted vests are all the rage on Instagram, and people have been touting their ability to help give you a harder workout, prevent bone loss, and maintain muscle strength. A five-year study found that weighted vest plus jumping exercises maintains hip bone mineral density by preventing significant bone loss in older postmenopausal women.

Increasing your body weight makes you work harder as you walk or do a workout and challenges your cardio and musculoskeletal systems. I like the idea of them, but there is a caveat: It can change the gravity and center of mass for women, which alters biomechanics. Because it's our lumbar spine and hips that need the extra load, and not our shoulders, some people prefer a weighted belt, which keeps the center of gravity where it needs to be. If you like your vest, just make sure you're not overdoing it with the weights to the point that you compromise your form and balance.

Personally, I love mine and I'm osteopenic. The decision to use a weighted vest or weight belt, though, is highly individual. If you are already exercising and fit, this is a different type of decision than for someone who is frail, prone to falls, and already osteoporitic. When in doubt, speak to your healthcare team. Factors that go into choosing a vest:

- Personal preferences: What feels best on your shoulders; this goes along with not using too much weight at first. I typically recommend 10 percent of your body weight, but some suggest lower numbers to start with.
- Cost: They are pretty reasonable, but range widely from thirty to a hundred dollars
- If you have a personal history of falls, osteoporosis, a weak core, or back injury, this is probably not for you. I would recommend you discuss with your medical provider first.

When first using a weighted vest, you may need to slow down your speed, if you are using it while walking outside or on a treadmill. I typically walk on my treadmill at 3.8 miles per hour with a weighted vest and 4.2 miles per hour without it.

Vibration plates (whole-body vibration training, or WBVT)

Dr. Terry Wahls, author of *The Wahls Protocol*, introduced me to these plates a few years ago, and I have never looked back. But first, what are they? They are motorized platforms that you can either stand, sit, or plank on as they vibrate back and forth. The transmission of this mechanical vibration triggers a tonic vibration reflex (TVR), a complex spinal and supraspinal neurophysiological reaction. This TVR can in turn activate muscles and improve physical performance. When stimulated by vibration, tactile feedback and intrinsic sensations help to control posture stability. WBVT plates are gaining popularity in helping with circulation, but they have also been shown to have positive effects on all parts of the human body, improving strength, balance, and functional mobility, reducing oxygen intake, as well as increasing blood flow, bone mineral density, cardiopulmonary function, and vascular function in older adults.

Patients who otherwise might not be ideal candidates for other types of exercise, such as the elderly, can typically safely engage in WBVT—it will even help decrease the likelihood of falls.

A vibration plate is a great add-on option to strength training, and zone 2 or flexibility work. (I like the Lifepro brand, but there are many options available at different price points.)

Caution: If you have a history of degenerative disk diseases, chronic back issues, or serious mobility problems, check with your healthcare provider first.

One last thing: Exercise helps support cognition and brain health. All movement boosts our health, but short periods of high-intensity resistance training and high-intensity cardio exercise significantly help attenuate cognitive decline. You know what else exercise does? It will inevitably improve your sleep. And for more ways to optimize your sleep, turn the page to the next chapter.

Chapter Summary

1. Keep moving. Just keep moving.
2. Musculoskeletal syndrome of menopause is a real thing, as is sarcopenia.
3. Exercise—specifically cardio—helps your gut microbiome stay healthy.
4. With few exceptions, everyone should be strength training.

References for this chapter can be found on my website: cynthiathurlow.com/themenopausegut-references

Chapter 8

Sleep like a Baby

"I used to sleep like a baby," Kristine, a forty-seven-year-old orthodontist, told me, "but now it is a struggle to even get a few hours before it's two or three in the morning and I am struggling to fall back to sleep, only to be woken up by my alarm clock."

Sound like you? Nearly every woman will experience some degree of sleep disturbances at this stage in her life. Women are more likely to suffer from sleep disorders than men as we advance in age, from 16 to 47 percent at perimenopause and up to 60 percent after the menopause transition. It is something you may have never really struggled with before, but all of a sudden, it's blaringly obvious that sleep has become a second job. Don't despair—even though the stats are stacked against us, there are many things you can do to offset the middlepause effects on getting enough good-quality, restful sleep. It also depends on what stage we are at in menopause: A study using data from the National Health Interview Survey found that sleep complaints tend to vary based on your menopausal stage. Perimenopausal women were more likely to sleep less than seven hours a night and report poor sleep quality, while menopausal women were more likely to have trouble falling asleep and staying asleep.

Here is the paradox: As we get older, it is even more important to get enough sleep. But with the changes in progesterone and estrogen levels, it's hard to get a good night's sleep. What's a middle-aged woman to do?

Let's find out what exactly sleep does for us, and then we'll take a deeper dive into how we can get more of it.

What Is Sleep, Exactly?

It's our body's shutdown mode. While our bodies rest and relax, many internal mechanisms begin their important work of needed repair and restoration of our systems, like our immune and endocrine systems. It is also a time when the brain is highly active.

Sleep Stages

There are four stages of sleep, broken into two main categories: non–rapid eye movement (NREM) and rapid eye movement (REM) sleep. (Did an R.E.M. song just pop into your head?)

1. **Light sleep:** The stage from being awake to falling asleep. This is just a few minutes, but your heart rate and breathing slow.
2. **Deeper light sleep:** You fall into a sleep but can still be woken up easily. Your body temperature drops, and your breathing and heart rates continue to slow. This lasts anywhere from ten to twenty-five minutes.
3. **Non-REM or deep sleep:** This is the first stage of deep sleep, when brain waves known as delta waves begin to emerge. It's also the sleep stage when your body begins to repair itself and shores up the immune system. This stage is crucial to feeling rested the next day. Most important, our brains are less metabolically active during this deep sleep, which allows for constriction of blood vessels and turning on the glymphatic system, our body's waste-removal process. If the glymphatic system doesn't work properly—due to poor sleep, aging, or brain injury—toxic proteins can build up, leading to memory loss, cognitive decline, and neurodegenerative diseases.

4. **REM sleep:** This is sleep's sweet spot. It's the most restorative period, as it helps our brains grow, develop, and learn. It's important for creativity and problem-solving, it processes emotional memories, and it helps maintain emotional awareness. If you don't get enough REM sleep, you can start to have memory and attention problems and mood issues, and there is an increased risk of disease.

A full sleep cycle—stages 1 through 4—should last about 90 to 120 minutes and typically repeats 4 to 6 times during the night. If you are not getting 7 to 9 hours of high-quality sleep every night, it is costing you your health. You can't roll over sleep hours—meaning, you can't make up for lost sleep the next night, on the weekends, or on vacation or when the stars and moon align. So, it's time to get our rest, and get it consistently.

What Happens When You Don't Get Enough Good Sleep?

Because sleep is when deep body-repair work is done, not giving our bodies enough time to do so can result in serious health problems. Studies show that even one night of sleeplessness will affect your focus and ability to think and make decisions clearly, not to mention leaving you feeling tired all day. Physical consequences add up if you don't get adequate sleep in the long term: It can weaken your immune system and make you more susceptible to viruses and disease; it can mess with your metabolism and increase your risk of diabetes and obesity; it can affect your cardiovascular system, increasing chances of a heart attack and stroke; and it can affect your mood, possibly leading you down the road to depression and anxiety.

You know what else you do if you don't get enough sleep? You feel hungry. You gravitate toward unhealthy food choices. I recall a time during perimenopause when I had a horrific string of sleepless nights despite trying everything. It is no surprise that I started craving salty, sugary foods. One example: Around Halloween, I found myself inhaling mini Reese's Peanut Butter Cups that were left over from trick-or-treating. I didn't have two or three. I had twenty! The cravings worsened how I felt and contributed to energy dips throughout the day. I knew what I was doing was bad for me, so I became more diligent about sleep hygiene and got serious about prioritizing sleep over my never-ending to-do list and those super-early workouts I used to insist on doing.

How Does Menopause Change Our Sleep?

Let's dig a little deeper into what is going on with our sleep as we transition from perimenopause into menopause. First, we get a roller-coaster ride of less circulating progesterone. Low levels of this hormone, like in early perimenopause, can show up as anxiety, depression, irritability, and insomnia. This loss of progesterone puts a greater strain on our adrenal glands, which also produce progesterone. Because the adrenals are part of our stress-management system, the hormonal changes in perimenopause can drive a decline in stress resilience, so that we can't cope with stress like we used to. Increased stress and poor coping can make perimenopause symptoms worse. This, in turn, can further exacerbate poor sleep quality.

Second, we experience changes in our circadian rhythm due to shifts in estrogen. Because estrogen is responsible for helping to coordinate our circadian clock, we'll get fluctuating levels of estrogen in the beginning and middle of perimenopause, and then in later stages, even less estrogen will exacerbate insomnia issues.

There's also less circulating melatonin, which is not just a sleep hormone, it is a master antioxidant, and our bodies are making less endogenous melatonin as we're getting older. We're less able to deal with stress. This doesn't mean that we are incapable. It just means that as we are having all these hormonal fluctuations, with less circulating progesterone, our adrenal glands are stepping in to help provide extra support. And in many instances, women, whether it's due to chronic stress, overtraining, not getting enough sleep, eating highly inflammatory foods, being in a toxic relationship or toxic job, or just being unhappy in their current stage of life, become less stress-resilient—and that can also impact sleep.

Another hormone impacted by aging is growth hormone (GH). GH impacts cell repair, muscle recovery, and tissue regeneration and can lead to bone-density issues; it also has neuroprotective effects, supports memory, focus, and learning, and stimulates collagen production, keeping our skin firm and hydrated.

When there is a lower level of circulating estrogen, like in the later stages of perimenopause and menopause, it impacts GH secretion and how our cells respond to it. A decline in GH secretion is called somatopause.

Around age fifty, GH secretion is reduced, leading to significant changes in body composition, such as reduced muscle mass. It also leads to lower energy and slows cellular repair and muscle recovery. GH reduction can lead to bone loss (likely exacerbated by low estrogen) as well as a loss of its neuroprotective effects, because it supports memory, focus, and learning.

In terms of sleep, because GH plays a crucial role in promoting quality sleep, particularly deep, slow-wave sleep during the first half of the night, lower levels can lead to disrupted sleep patterns and increased insomnia in postmenopausal women.

OBSTRUCTIVE SLEEP APNEA (OSA)

Menopausal females have a greater likelihood of developing OSA, a sleep disorder in which a person's breathing repeatedly stops and starts. The rise of susceptibility is due to changes in, you guessed it, estrogen and progesterone. These hormones help keep our airway muscles strong, and their decline makes the airway more prone to collapse during sleep, which can lead to periods of apnea (pauses in breathing), disrupted sleep, and oxygen deprivation. OSA can also impair deep sleep and the functioning of our glymphatic system. If the glymphatic system is impaired, it increases the buildup of toxins that may increase our risk of Alzheimer's, memory loss, and brain fog. OSA also contributes to high blood pressure, heart disease, poor metabolic health, and an overall worsening of hot flashes.

If you suspect you might suffer from sleep apnea, I suggest going to your provider and seeing what your options are. They may suggest seeing a specialist who can do some polysomnography testing (sleep study); depending on the results, they may recommend weight loss, HRT, or a CPAP (continuous positive airway pressure), which is the standard of care, or BiPAP (bilevel positive airway pressure), which is typically reserved for those who do not respond favorably to CPAP or have severe COPD and/or OSA.

The Gut-Sleep Connection

Growing evidence suggests that the gut microbiome can influence sleep quality and vice versa. Good microbiome diversity equals good sleep, period.

Poor sleep disrupts the gut microbiome and that can show up as bloating, gas, diarrhea, or constipation. We have to be in our parasympathetic (rest and repose) nervous system to feel "safe" to poop, so when stressed, many women stop going. And women who already had digestive issues during menopause may find their symptoms worsen with poor sleep. Poor sleep can also lead to high cortisol, which can further disrupt the gut microbiome and potentially lead to leaky gut (due to alterations in immune function). Sleep deprivation can affect appetite hormones, leading to increased appetite and unhealthy food choices, which further influence gut health.

It's important to note that those who are at greatest risk for the sequelae of sleep issues are people who are at a lower socioeconomic status, with a lower educational level and lower income, and without a supportive partner. It makes sense that if you are burdened with financial stressors and an unsupportive partner, it can make navigating this transitional period quite challenging. These additional stressors can exacerbate symptoms, including vasomotor symptoms, which can result in poor sleep.

Kathy was one of these people who had trouble sleeping. At age sixty, she was well into menopause, and someone very close to her had just died. Overcome with grief, she had trouble falling and staying asleep. She was unmotivated to eat and take care of herself. She became clinically depressed. When she first came to see me, I referred her to a local psychologist to develop effective strategies to process her loss while we worked on improving nutrition. We adjusted her supplements and included Seriphos, which helps with blunting the effects of cortisol in the short term; Relora, an adaptogenic herb that nourishes the adrenals; and ashwagandha. She also added about a third to a half cup of high-quality carbs (sweet potato, squash, lentils) to her dinner. I recommended some deep breathing exercises and an Apollo Neuro device to help calm her fight-or-flight response. With diligent support from friends, family, her psychologist, and my team, we had her sleeping better within three weeks. She was still grieving—nothing can help alleviate that except time—but at least she was well rested.

Healthy Sleep Also Means Healthy Weight

I often tell my patients that sleep is critically important, especially for those trying to lose weight. A study published in the *Canadian Medical Association Journal* showed that sleep deprivation is directly related to an inability to lose weight, meaning you will not lose the stubborn weight if you are not getting adequate sleep. Peak growth hormone is secreted at night during sleep. Remember, it helps your body heal and supports the development of lean muscle mass, but we start producing less of it as we age—so prioritizing high-quality sleep is crucial. This secretion isn't going to happen unless you get into a deep sleep. If you are waking up between two and four a.m., you aren't getting into the deep sleep you need to lose weight and support your health.

GETTING UP AT NIGHT TO PEE?

Have you noticed that you have been waking up at night to use the bathroom? You are not alone on this either: Nearly 90 percent of women in menopause experience nocturia, which is waking at night to urinate, relative specifically to the loss of estradiol, which directly impacts bladder capacity.

Getting up multiple times a night may actually induce anatomical and physiological changes in the bladder, and it can impact a reduction in functional bladder capacity. So, what all of that is saying is, in menopause, that loss of estrogen—if you're not doing HRT—will just exacerbate and magnify these issues. Your body is working against some of these normal physiologic mechanisms. Hormone replacement therapy can help with this. If you are struggling, I encourage you to discuss it with your internist and/or GYN.

Dos and Don'ts for Optimal Sleep

I ask all my clients to abide by the philosophy of *good, better, best*. I find that sometimes we have to do the best we can with what we have at the time. There may be nights when you don't have the best sleep, and that's OK; not everyone is going to sleep like a "bug in a rug" all the time. We just don't want it to become a pattern.

The following are healthy sleep dos and don'ts. Don't feel like you have to do *everything* on this list; if you can only start implementing a few, that is good, too.

During the Day

Do

1. **Get sunlight exposure early in the morning.** This helps to suppress melatonin and increase cortisol to get our day started. Do this within the first two hours of waking and without sunglasses. If you want to get up earlier, start by adding light in the morning within twenty minutes of waking. This will suppress melatonin and increase cortisol.

2. **Limit caffeine** to about twelve ounces, especially if you are sensitive (a slow metabolizer). Caffeine offsets the receptors for a neurotransmitter by-product called adenosine. It tricks your brain into thinking you're not tired by covering up those "slow-down" signals. But when the caffeine wears off, all that adenosine is still there, so you feel even more sleepy. I like to remind patients that caffeine has a half-life of four to eight hours depending on the individual, so it is important to limit or eliminate it after twelve p.m. If you find that it is particularly challenging to limit caffeine in the morning, it may be a sign that your cortisol is dysregulated. I find that my patients with the lowest morning cortisol are typically addicted to caffeine to help with energy throughout the day.

3. **Do something physical.** Our bodies were designed to move. When we break a sweat and are active during our awake hours, it helps our brains understand the difference between activity and rest. It's essential to align our body with our circadian rhythm. Going for a walk, washing the car, and playing with pets or kids during daylight hours also help to establish this.

4. **Work out in the morning if you can.** A study at Appalachian State University in Boone, North Carolina, found that morning

workouts are ideal if we want to get the best sleep at night. Researchers tracked sleep patterns of participants who worked out at different times and found that those who exercised at seven a.m. slept longer and had a deeper sleep cycle than the other groups—up to 75 percent more time in deep sleep. Exercise is great, but if you exercise too late, you may stay up later. Exercise raises your body temperature and gives you a burst of energy that could hinder your ability to fall asleep. It's equally important to be active throughout the day, aiming for five thousand to ten thousand steps per day.

5. **Eat enough and earlier.** If you are practicing intermittent fasting and OMAD (one meal a day), you might not be consuming enough macronutrients. If you are truly hungry, this is going to disrupt your sleep. You want stable blood sugar throughout the night. Your food choices should focus on protein and healthy fats. Add in carbohydrates from starchy vegetables and low-glycemic fruits. Also, you don't want to have your meals within three hours of bedtime, in order to avoid the negative impacts of digestion on sleep quality.

6. **Filter your air.** I'm a huge fan of air-filtration systems (Levoit is a nice brand) or even using plants in the home. NASA studied about a dozen popular varieties of ornamental indoor plants to determine their effectiveness in removing several key pollutants associated with indoor air pollution and found that living plants are very efficient at absorbing contaminants in the air. Examples are spider plants, Boston ferns, and English ivy.

7. **Support your gut microbiome.** An unhealthy gut microbiome influences the health of our neurotransmitters, including serotonin, which is the building block for melatonin. Estrogen plays a crucial role in modulating our serotonin receptors, and when our

estrogen fluctuates, the sensitivity and responsiveness of our serotonin receptors can also be impacted.

8. **Eat organic fruits and veggies** to reduce your exposure to pesticides and herbicides (see page 121). I know organic is more expensive, but this will help your gut health and in turn your sleep—and you know what? They just. Taste. Better. This is one place where the money will be well spent.

9. **Get your hugs!** We know that oxytocin helps to naturally lower cortisol and can help induce sleep. We can get these effects through hugging and cuddling, holding hands, massage, orgasm, connecting with loved ones, meditation, and even petting our animals. Enough said—connection, connection, connection is so important!

10. **Rule out sleep apnea** and get a polysonography test, if needed.

11. **Look into HRT**, especially progesterone, estrogen, and melatonin. (HRT will be discussed in chapter 10.)

12. **Take supplements.** We will speak at length about supplements in chapter 12, but for now, consider these for sleep: myo-inositol, magnesium, l-theanine, glycine, and adaptogens like ashwagandha and magnolia bark, to name just a few.

13. **Drink tea.** Some teas, like chamomile, can be beneficial at night. Also, emerging research on certain bacteria, like *Bifidobacterium longum* 1714, shows that they may improve sleep, reduce stress, and even improve cognitive function.

Around Bedtime

Do

1. **Take magnesium.** After all my years working in cardiology as a nurse practitioner, I'm savvy with electrolytes, and magnesium is one that most of us are deficient in. Our bodies use up this nutrient quickly as a way to combat stress, and having adequate magnesium levels helps your body rest in a restorative state. I like both oral magnesium and transdermal (absorbed through the skin). I also recommend a pure magnesium oil spray or lotion from a company called Ancient Minerals. This transdermal spray helps replenish your magnesium stores, and there is a sensitive-skin option for those who are more likely to react to topical forms of magnesium. (We will discuss magnesium in greater detail in chapter 12, but I recommend taking oral magnesium daily as well as using transdermal options a few days per week.)

2. **Go to bed early and consistently.** The ideal time to hit the sack is by ten p.m., as this aligns with the natural rise in melatonin. There has been a lot of research on night-shift workers (ER nurses and doctors, security guards, night factory workers, etc.), and the results are consistent in showing a significant impact on the increased risk of sleep disorders and health problems—so much so that the International Agency for Research on Cancer has now classified overnight shift work as a carcinogen. This chronic sleep pattern can also put someone at risk for breast cancer, diabetes, and poor metabolic health.

3. **Meditate to manage your stress.** Does your mind constantly race when you're trying to fall asleep? Counting sheep suddenly becomes counting all the things on your to-do list? Try to empty your mind and focus on breathing. If you need a guided meditation, you can try that, too. The app Headspace has a bunch of

great ones, and I have a friend who swears by listening to Harry Styles read her a bedtime story on Calm. There is also meditative music specifically for inducing sleep on Spotify and other music platforms. I love guided meditations to help bring on sleep. Get on a PEMF mat (see chapter 9), or put your legs up a wall to relax before sleep.

4. **Turn down the thermostat.** Studies have found that the optimal room temperature for sleep is anywhere from sixty to sixty-eight degrees, which is even more important with our temperature regulation being disrupted in middle age. Understanding how the HPA axis is impacted at this midlife transition is important. Research suggests that you can induce better sleep by taking a hot bath or shower sixty to ninety minutes before bedtime; I don't do this every night, but it can be quite effective when I do. The warm bath or shower increases vasodilation, whereby blood moves from our core to our extremities. This then promotes a drop in our core body temperature and signals to our brain that it is time to go to bed.

5. **Adjust to the dark.** If you want to go to bed later, expose yourself to more light in the afternoon to help postpone bedtime. You also want to make sure that you're exposed to darkness before falling asleep; otherwise, light exposure will suppress melatonin.

6. **Darken your room.** You don't have to live like a vampire, but having a dark room will help you get to sleep faster and stay asleep, as it helps melatonin production and sets that circadian clock to sleep mode. I'm a huge fan of silk sleeping masks: They help block out all the light, and it is such a simple way of supporting sleep.

7. **Avoid drinking alcohol.** Women metabolize alcohol differently than men. Because we have less lean mass and more body fat,

we process alcohol faster. This means that after a woman and a man of the same weight drink the same amount of alcohol, the woman's blood alcohol concentration (the amount of alcohol in the blood) will tend to be higher, putting her at greater risk for harm. Alcohol is incredibly disruptive to REM sleep and dysregulates our blood sugar, leading to vasomotor symptoms, hot flashes, and poor dietary choices the following day. There is no amount of alcohol that is benign. Bottom line: Alcohol is a greater contributor to interrupted sleep than almost anything else. If you do drink alcohol in the evening, follow it up with equal amounts of water, and do follow your regular nighttime routine.

8. **Avoid exposing yourself to blue light.** Blue light—a wavelength found in all our electronics—suppresses the production of sleepytime melatonin. Researchers at Brigham and Women's Hospital in Boston found that the use of light-emitting electronic devices in the hours before bedtime can adversely impact overall health, alertness, and our circadian clock. The study showed that readers who read on an iPad took longer to fall asleep and had shorter REM sleep compared with test subjects who were assigned a physical book. The iPad readers also secreted less melatonin and were more tired than the book readers, even if they slept for eight hours. If you must, wear blue-light-blocking glasses or download an app like f.lux (for Mac), which eliminates problematic blue light on devices at specific intervals. The same goes for watching TV, which emits blue light. It is not quieting your mind; it is only exciting it. Try going to sleep by reading a book, the old-fashioned kind with paper pages.

9. **Smell your way to sleep.** The connection between our sense of smell and our brains is strong and can have a profound impact on our stress response. Our brain can often associate pleasant smells with calming effects, essentially activating the "rest and digest"

function of the parasympathetic nervous system, leading to physiological changes like decreased heart rate and improved digestion.

10. **Consider HRT.** This, with other interventions, can be a true game changer for sleep quality. No one should suffer with poor-quality sleep. I find that progesterone is very helpful for falling asleep and even a bit sedating, and estrogen can be helpful for *staying* asleep. Obviously, there are many considerations, but please have a discussion with your provider about the appropriateness of this intervention.

11. **Avoid becoming dependent on melatonin.** Yes, melatonin is a natural sleep aid, and I suggest using it if you are going through a stressful time. But it should not be the only way to get you to sleep.

12. **Avoid late-night snacks.** Ideally, finish eating three hours before bedtime. You don't want those circadian clock receptors in the GI tract triggered if you are trying to unwind for the night. Plan your meals accordingly so that the last one has plenty of time to digest before bedtime. If you eat too close to bedtime, it will blunt the secretion of melatonin, and your cortisol will increase to help process your food.

13. **Stop pushing the four thirty a.m. workout.** Yes, I love a good workout, but I don't think you should win a gold star for doing so day after day, especially after limited sleep. You will see greater results from prioritizing rest, recovery, and sleep than you will from pushing your body to its limits.

Sleep Gadget Hacks

With sleep being so crucial to our health, it's only natural that companies and experts are always tinkering with contraptions to help people get more z's. Check out the latest innovations that I have recommended to my clients:

Elemind is a headband-like device that has EEG sensors and sends acoustic pulses to interfere with alpha brain waves and help you get to sleep faster—and put you back to sleep if you wake up. Please note it does require a subscription and is considered to be a luxury, but it's a fun one!

The Oura Ring, my personal favorite, is a health-tracking device; it helps record heart rate, heart rate variability (HRV), blood oxygen levels, and body temperature. While many use it to track their physical activity during the day, it is particularly good if you need to monitor your sleep, as it will provide in-depth data about your sleep stages and even give you a "sleep score." I really like my patients to be mindful of patterns with regard to REM and deep sleep metrics, aiming for ninety minutes of each per night.

Chill pads and pillows: I know I am not the only one who has woken up in a pool of sweat while in perimenopause or menopause. It's a natural response to lower estrogen levels making the hypothalamus think the body is running hot. This can also be problematic with blood sugar dysregulation. If you are not mindful of macros, you can see fluctuations in blood glucose driving vasomotor symptoms, as well. These mattress pads, pillows, and blankets can cool your body temperature while you sleep. (It won't help with your husband's snoring, unfortunately.)

Naps

If you are a nap person, I recommend keeping naps short and earlier in the day. During menopause, naps, especially later in the day, can negatively impact overall sleep patterns by disrupting your circadian rhythm and making it harder to fall asleep at night, potentially leading to further sleep disturbances like insomnia due to the hormonal fluctuations experienced during this time; therefore, it's recommended to keep naps short and early in the afternoon. If you need a nap, keep it to fifteen to twenty minutes—I refer to these as power naps. I tend to reserve these for days when I've either had a shorter night of sleep than usual (with traveling, etc.) or if I'm starting to feel like I may be getting sick.

WHAT IF I'M A SELF-PROCLAIMED NIGHT OWL?

Far be it from me to tell you to go against your chronotype—your natural inclination for when you feel most awake and most sleepy. Think of your chronotype as your body's own internal clock personality. Whether you are an early bird or a night owl is influenced by our circadian rhythms. They work on a twenty-four-hour schedule and influence our sleep-wake cycles, body temperature, when hormones are released, how alert we are, how much energy we have, when we want to exercise, and so on. Our chronotypes are also influenced by genetics, age, and life stage factors. You may notice that teenagers tend to stay up later and sleep in versus older adults, who tend to wake up earlier, eat earlier, and go to bed earlier—all of which is influenced by life stage, genetics, and lifestyle.

Advice usually tips to the early bird's favor on sleep patterns, but the research does show that even for a night owl, there are things you can do to support your sleep quality, like being mindful of the cortisol triggers that may keep you up later than you want to be. Also know there may be some health risks involved: One study shows that evening chronotypes in both peri- and postmenopause have a risk factor for the development of diabetes.

Still awake? Good. Let's find out how we can get rid of some of that stress that keeps us up at night.

Chapter Summary

1. Prioritize sleep like your life depends on it, because it does.
2. Manage your stress proactively throughout the day to help support sleep.
3. Get early sunlight in the morning to help suppress melatonin and raise your cortisol.
4. Don't eat close to bedtime, and turn off that phone.
5. Consider HRT and/or supplementation.

References for this chapter can be found on my website: cynthiathurlow.com/themenopausegut-references

Chapter 9

Stressed Out

"I'm so stressed out I can't see straight."

Jessica, forty-seven, a manager at a marketing firm and a mom of two, came to see me out of utter frustration. As a member of the sandwich generation, she was busy at work, raising kids, and now taking care of her parents. In addition, she was having a myriad of signs suggestive of perimenopause, such as irregular cycles, heavy bleeding, and worsening premenstrual symptoms (mood swings, fatigue, breast tenderness). She also noticed her stress levels going through the roof. She was irritable and had difficulty concentrating, feeling overwhelmed at both work and home. These physically manifested as frequent tension headaches, neck and shoulder stiffness, and digestive issues (bloating and acid reflux). She also had trouble falling and staying asleep. She'd always had stress in her life, but this was "next level" for her. She confessed to me, "Between work's tight deadlines, my teen kids needing my attention, and my parents needing help with doctor's appointments, I'm really feeling totally overwhelmed. And then, on top of all that, I am supposed to just 'deal' with these perimenopause issues? No thanks!"

Let's be clear, no one can really avoid stress—it's in our everyday lives, whether it's dealing with a sick baby or bad traffic on the way home from work. And unfortunately, the estrogen and progesterone fluctuations during perimenopause can impact mood-regulating neurotransmitters like serotonin and dopamine, which can create a feeling of worsening anxiety and being "stressed out" during this time, exacerbating any psychosocial, physical, and emotional issues we may be going through.

We can usually fight off stress with our own inner resilience and natural defenses, but when stress becomes chronic—when there is no let-up in the assaults our body takes—it creates a continuous release of adrenaline and cortisol. This constant hyper-reaction can lead to harmful effects on overall health, including an increased risk of developing serious illnesses like heart disease and diabetes. Chronic stress can also take a toll on mental health, making it difficult to manage when our mood takes a dive and our focus dissipates into thin air. Studies show that women are much more susceptible to depression and other mood disorders in middlepause. For example, the risk for new-onset depression in women without a history of depression increases twofold during perimenopause, an effect that is exacerbated by exposure to early childhood trauma.

Taking steps to manage stress is important not only for feeling better day-to-day but also for supporting long-term health and well-being. Otherwise, many compounding physical and physiological issues can flood in. I speak from both personal and professional experience here: Women who navigate this part of their lives tend to do best if they are proactively integrating stress-management activities into their day-to-day life (and five to ten minutes of meditation once a week won't cut it).

What is the difference between acute and chronic stress? If the enormity of stressors we face keeps us in a perpetual fight-or-flight situation, with our sympathetic nervous system continually activated, over time, it can wear our bodies down, elevate cortisol, and negatively impact our health. As Dr. Sara Gottfried, bestselling author of *The Autoimmune Cure*, says, "Stress can be a vague term, and that makes it difficult to neutralize."

We'll look into the significance of early childhood stress and trauma a bit later in the chapter, as it has been a grossly overlooked contributor to chronic stress and can put women at greater risk for a slew of health issues during the menopausal transition. But first, let's see what else all that extra stress can do to our bodies.

How Does Stress Impact Our Gut Health?

We talked a lot about stress in chapter 1, and while we know that having some can be beneficial and can make us stronger and more resilient, most of us have too much stress, too often, and too consistently. These day-in, day-out high stress levels negatively impact not only our health but also our gut microbiome. Then we throw middle age in there and all this can lead to a reduction in microbial diversity, which has a huge domino effect on our body, leading to hyper-permeability (leaky gut), which can then lead to chronic inflammation and susceptibility to opportunistic infections (dysbiosis and more). Furthermore, it can impact our mood, as well as metabolism and weight gain.

Additionally, stress can also alter immune function, especially if that stress was experienced early in life and was significant: Studies show that childhood stressors may elicit long-lasting immune consequences and increase the risk of developing stress-related disorders later in life. Chronic stress can also negatively impact key mood-improving neurotransmitters, like GABA, serotonin, and dopamine, that are produced by healthy gut bacteria. Chronic stress begets more stress and strain on our bodies and health. All this is why it is important to diligently work on managing our stress.

Cortisol Changes Also Factor In as We Age

We talked about cortisol in chapter 4, but because this is a major stress hormone, here we are again. Cortisol has been with us since humans stood erect. It was a lifesaver back in the day when we had real, immediate threats to our lives (like a bear or tiger chasing us). But today, when you're stressed out, your body perceives it is under attack and produces more cortisol to give you strength and energy to defend yourself. Your body doesn't differentiate between running from a rabid animal and being stressed out dealing with traffic trying to get to work or your children's school play.

When the threat passes, cortisol levels typically fall back closer to baseline, and your body should return to its normal state, thanks to an opposing system—the parasympathetic nervous system (PNS). Ideally, it takes over and calms your body down after the "danger" has passed. But with the onset of middlepause, cortisol, our stress hormone, and GABA, our calming neurotransmitter, impact stress levels significantly due to hormonal fluctuations, particularly the decline in estrogen and progesterone. These changes can lead to higher baseline cortisol levels, increased stress sensitivity, and difficulty regulating the stress response.

What does this lead to? Many, many women reaching their middlepause years, like Jessica, are in a state of perpetual fight-or-flight mode due to chronic stress. That is not an ideal way to spend the rest of your life. We sometimes refer to this as sympathetic dominance, that chronic stress cycle that can erode our health substantially.

What can we do about it? A lot, actually. There are many stress-lowering activities and therapies we can do (which we cover later in this chapter), but first let's figure out that blurry line where manageable stress turns into unmanageable stress.

Can We Measure Stress?

We have an old saying in medicine: You can't monitor what you do not measure. Quantifying stress is complex because stress is both a physical and psychological experience, but there are several approaches—both subjective and objective—that can help measure it. HRV (heart rate variability) is one of the best measures. This refers to the variation of time between consecutive heartbeats. Measured in milliseconds, it is influenced by two parts of our autonomic nervous system (ANS): The sympathetic nervous system (SNS) activates the fight, flight, freeze, or fawn response, increasing heart rate and reducing variability, and the parasympathetic nervous system (PNS) governs the rest-and-digest state, slowing heart rate and increasing variability. (Think of SNS as the gas pedal in a car, accelerating the stress response, while the PNS acts like the brake pedal, slowing the stress response.)

A healthy heart does not beat like a clock ticks; instead, it adapts to the body's needs by varying the time between beats. If the system is in more of a fight-or-flight mode (sympathetic dominant), the variation between subsequent heartbeats tends to be lower. If the system is in a more relaxed state (parasympathetic dominant), the variation between beats may be higher.

These fluctuations are undetectable except with specialized devices. The gold standard for a true reading is the old-fashioned electrocardiogram (ECG or EKG). However, I'm a realist and recognize that most people are not signing up for EKGs on the regular, nor do they want to be hooked up to an EKG machine 24-7, so using wearable devices is a great way to easily assess how your HRV is being impacted day-to-day by your lifestyle. HRV can be tracked in real time to observe stress responses during specific events (e.g., a stressful meeting) or recovery phases (e.g., after meditation or exercise) using devices like smartwatches, fitness trackers, or heart rate monitors. (The best gadgets are made by companies like Garmin, Fitbit, Whoop, and Oura Ring.)

A high HRV (above 70 milliseconds) = lower stress. A high HRV suggests strong parasympathetic activity, indicating the body is relaxed and resilient to stressors. People with high HRV tend to recover more quickly from stress.

A low HRV (below 50 milliseconds) = higher stress. When you're under stress, your SNS dominates, leading to a more consistent, rapid heart rate and lower HRV. Chronic stress can result in persistently low HRV, indicating that the body is in a prolonged state of fight-or-flight.

People with a higher HRV score are generally in better health, less stressed, and happier, while those with lower HRV are more stressed and tired, or may be in poor health. (Most of my patients struggle with chronic over-activation of the SNS and therefore have low HRV.) Low HRV is considered a sign of current or a predictor of future health problems because it shows that your body is less resilient and struggles to handle changing situations. I also see variations in HRV around travel, significant changes in altitude, during a woman's menstrual cycle, or even when someone is getting sick. In these scenarios, you may experience lowered

HRV, poorer sleep quality, and higher heart rate, so these trackers can be helpful in providing input on multiple lifestyle modalities.

In addition to measuring HRV, there are other ways of measuring your stress levels. I am a fan of surveys and questionnaires, journaling, measuring cortisol (via serum, urine, or saliva), and checking vital signs, sleep habits, physical activity, and more. If you are in a university or other academic setting, you may even participate in imaging (fMRI) or monitoring brain electrical activity (EEG). Surveys, questionnaires, and journaling can be done independently, although some mental health professionals utilize these tools in their practices. You can also refer to chapter 11 for more lab tests that can be done through a licensed healthcare provider.

When Is Stress Actually Traumatic?

When does normal daily stress become something more serious, beyond our control? Not all stress equates to trauma, but our perception of stressful circumstances has a huge impact if we experience a traumatic event(s). Dr. Gabor Maté, author of the groundbreaking book on trauma *The Myth of Normal*, refers to trauma as a wound: It is not what happens to you; it's what happens inside you as a result of what happened to you, and that trauma is a scarring that makes you less able to appropriately respond to acute or chronic stress. This was a big revelation for me: I was taught that trauma is big-T—rape, murder, suicide—and it was only later that I realized little-T trauma was equally impactful. Divorce, illness, job loss. So it's not surprising that it has been reported that 90 percent of Americans have experienced at least one traumatic event in their lifetime—the difference is how our bodies react to them. Some may come away from the experience OK; others may develop a long-term condition called post-traumatic stress disorder (PTSD). Demographics do come into play for increasing risk of PTSD, including gender (ticks up for being female), ethnicity (ticks up for African Americans), and socioeconomic status (more common in urban and lower socioeconomic areas). PTSD and depression following trauma exposure are more than twice as prevalent in women than men. Studies show that highest prevalence rates of PTSD in women occur in their early fifties, which coincides with the menopausal transition.

There has been very important research showing that traumas that happened in our childhood can affect us greatly (and many times unwittingly) as adults. Dr. Sara Gottfried has been on the forefront of observing the effects of childhood trauma and women navigating midlife and has written about how trauma dysregulates the PINE system—the psycho-immune-neuroendocrine network, a fancy phrase for the system between our brain and our bodies, including immune system, nervous system, and endocrine system, and how they all affect our physical, mental, and spiritual health. When this system becomes dysregulated, maladaptive, harmful, and pervasive issues can arise.

The long-term impact of sexual abuse is readily apparent in a twenty-three-year longitudinal study on multigenerational sexual abuse victims and their offspring, and the cumulative effect of violence and trauma. Research suggests that women who were sexually abused as children and go on to have children who are sexually abused will reach menopause earlier, at roughly age forty, which is almost nine years earlier than mothers who reported no abuse. *Nine* years.

How Childhood Experiences Affect Long-Term Health

It's only a relatively new concept that serious health problems can be tied to childhood traumatic events. The idea originally grew out of the work of Dr. Vincent Felitti, who was helping obese individuals lose weight in the mid-1980s. At the time a specialist in preventive medicine at San Diego's Kaiser Permanente, Dr. Felitti noticed that many of his patients had been abused as children, and weight gain was being used as a coping mechanism, or a "shield" against sexual attention or physical attack. Some had also used tobacco, alcohol, or drugs to cope. That original finding eventually led to the Adverse Childhood Experiences (ACE) Study, conducted by researchers at Kaiser Permanente and the Centers for Disease Control and Prevention (CDC) in the late 1990s. It studied the impact of specific negative childhood experiences and conditions on long-term health by grouping ACEs into three categories: abuse, neglect, and family/household challenges. In the study of more than seventeen thousand adults, researchers found that those with a high number of ACEs were at much greater risk for negative health outcomes like obesity, depression, sexually transmitted diseases, heart disease, broken bones, stroke, and even cancer. Those risks remained even when lifestyle choices like smoking and drinking were factored in. A high number of ACEs also affected life potential, such as lowering academic achievement and increasing the amount of sick time taken off from work. In addition, the study found that the impact of ACEs was cumulative: The more ACEs a person had, the more likely that person was to suffer from negative health outcomes. It can be predictive of future health issues, including depression, PTSD, autoimmune disease, and more, which we suspect is due to toxic stress on the person's developing brain in childhood that shows up later in middle age as chronic disease.

ACEs and Women

The CDC states that among US adults surveyed from 2011 to 2020, approximately two thirds reported at least one ACE, while one in six reported four or more ACEs. These were highest among women. The NIH reports that figure is 39 percent of females compared with 21 percent of males. That is nearly double the occurrence.

While research is young, there have been some solid studies that show the long-term effects of childhood trauma on physical health. The Study of Women's Health Across the Nation (SWAN) and the MsHeart/MsBrain studies are finding that midlife women who have experienced childhood physical, emotional, or sexual abuse are at greater risk of vascular disease, heart attack, stroke, and hot flashes than those without this history.

Childhood trauma has also been shown to contribute to a pro-inflammatory state and low cortisol in adulthood. For women who have experienced trauma, menopause can trigger a resurgence of emotional symptoms, often leading to intensified anxiety, depression, panic attacks, and even exacerbated physical symptoms like hot flashes and night sweats. Because of the sensitive nature of the body's stress response during menopause, the hormonal fluctuations during this time can reopen unresolved wounds from past trauma, potentially making it harder to manage these emotions. The changes in estrogen, dopamine, and serotonin can exacerbate mood changes, as these help with emotional regulation and mood stabilization. With these changes, it becomes challenging for women, even more so for those with a history of trauma.

Women who did not experience childhood trauma but later experienced neglect or abuse can also experience huge ramifications of PTSD and its increasing effects on middlepausal symptoms. Violence by an intimate partner against women is one of the most common forms of violence worldwide. The World Health Organization's *Global Status Report on Violence Prevention 2014*, for example, concluded that one in three women have been a victim of physical or sexual violence by an intimate partner at some point in their lifetime. The psychological toll of domestic violence is heavy: PTSD, depression, anxiety, substance misuse, and mental health issues. And the research supports that women who have experienced PTSD will likely experience more symptoms than their non-PTSD counterparts during the middlepause transition. Furthermore, the evolving research around intimate partner violence suggests that women who have experienced this degree of trauma (and subsequent chronic stress) have also profoundly impacted their HPA axis. The bottom line? Violence can accelerate reproductive aging.

While this all sounds scary and defeating, rest assured that there are many things to mitigate the past. But let's see where you stand first.

What's Your ACE Score?

As the science community does more work to quantify trauma, there is currently a simple measuring system for ACE, on a scale from 0 to 10. The ACE score is based on a questionnaire that asks about ten types of adverse experiences before the age of eighteen, categorized into three groups: abuse, neglect, and household challenges.

1. Did you feel that you didn't have enough to eat, had to wear dirty clothes, or had no one to protect or take care of you?
2. Did you lose a parent through divorce, abandonment, death, or other reason?
3. Did you live with anyone who was depressed, mentally ill, or attempted suicide?
4. Did you live with anyone who had a problem with drinking or using drugs, including prescription drugs?
5. Did your parents or adults in your home ever hit, punch, beat, or threaten to harm each other?
6. Did you live with anyone who went to jail or prison?
7. Did a parent or adult in your home ever swear at you, insult you, or put you down?
8. Did a parent or adult in your home ever hit, beat, kick, or physically hurt you in any way?
9. Did you feel that no one in your family loved you or thought you were special?
10. Did you experience unwanted sexual contact (such as fondling or oral/anal/vaginal intercourse/penetration)?

Full disclosure: I'm a 9. Yes, that is a very high score. My childhood was pretty traumatic, with physical and emotional abuse, emotional neglect, and a parent who was an alcoholic and also quite depressed. I do not share these details to garner sympathy, but mainly to share that I had significant childhood experiences, but through many years of therapy, close friendships, and a loving spouse and family, I was able to move beyond what I had experienced as a child.

I believe I have had multiple autoimmune conditions (all in remission) as a result of my childhood trauma, and I have to work extra hard at this stage of life because my autonomic nervous system tends to run in fight-or-flight mode. Remember Jessica from the top of this chapter? She had an ACE of 7. You are not alone if you took this test and realize that you have been harboring a lot of long-term trauma.

I know from all the work I did that there are many treatments and therapies that will help you with your stress levels—or if you had a high ACE score, with your unresolved trauma. Even at middlepause, it is *never* too late to heal yourself and make yourself more resilient against stress.

Ways to Lower Stress

Whether you are dealing with increased stress levels during menopause or wanting to mitigate your ACE scores, if you are currently dealing with an acute stressor, like the death of a loved one, a divorce, job loss, or move, every middle-aged woman needs multiple strategies to manage stress. I find, even in this day and age, that many women are largely disconnected from their bodies, so doing some internal exploration around what makes your body feel good versus more stressed is essential.

This list runs from the traditional (therapy) and basic (meditation, yoga) to more intense and experimental (MDMA-assisted therapies). If you feel you need a more experimental or progressive therapy than what you have readily available, connect with a mental health provider or your primary care provider to determine the best course of action for you.

I am a fan of using multiple treatments, but it is up to you. Everyone is different, and what works for your neighbor may not work for you. And by no means is this an exhaustive list of options; rather, they are some of my personal favorites and favorites of my clients. I find most of my patients do best with finding out (1) what they may be interested in, and (2) what they can afford. Simple exercises like breathwork, meditation, and yoga can be done at home and for free, but treatments like therapy, PEMF (pulsed electromagnetic field), and acupuncture involve a professional and/or equipment and therefore come at a cost. So read up on these therapies and decide what suits you and your budget best. The number one rule is to be proactive about it. If stress is a big factor in your life, you need to prioritize time for managing it. Everyone has five to ten minutes on a daily basis, so make it a habit for a better you.

Note: Before beginning any of these therapies, consult your internist or PCP to see if they are right for you and make sure you don't have any preexisting conditions that may be impacted.

Traditional Therapy

Sometimes just talking to someone and vocalizing your anxieties to an objective and impartial person can help enormously, so teaming up with a good mental health professional, psychiatrist, or psychologist is a great way to go if you are suffering with stress, anxiety, or PTSD. Methods vary—from psychotherapy to cognitive behavioral therapy (CBT)—and most have been well tested and proven effective. Some therapists take insurance, some don't. I know a lot of people who have gotten the best recommendations through friends and primary caregivers.

Yoga

With many physical and mental benefits, a yoga practice may be something that you can incorporate into your daily life and do as a supplement to another therapy. By combining postures to improve flexibility and strength, breathing exercises to relax, and meditation to focus, yoga can calm that important vagus nerve and lower stress levels. Studies show what ancient yogis have known for centuries: The practice can dampen the brain's stress response as well as help with the regulation of emotions. Your gut may benefit, too: Emerging research suggests that yoga may influence the gut–brain axis by balancing the diversity of gut microbiota. This balance is crucial for optimal digestive health and overall well-being.

There are so many online and streaming classes that are free—there really isn't a good reason not to at least try yoga. You may just have a hard time figuring out which is best for you. There are several types, including hatha, vinyasa, Ashtanga, and yin yoga; all have varying degrees of approach, some more meditative, others more athletic. Finding one that you like may feel like dating, but once you find one that suits you, it may just change your life. For stress reduction, I typically recommend avoiding the more intensive yoga practices, like Ashtanga, and sticking to yin, vinyasa, or even the delicious yoga nidra, a personal favorite.

Mindfulness Meditation

"Meditation" can scare some people off, as it may sound too woo-woo, but the practice is actually very simple. It's about being present and observing thoughts without judgment, for a specific time period. There is really no right or wrong way to do it. Researchers reviewed more than two hundred studies of mindfulness among healthy people and found mindfulness-based therapy was especially effective for reducing stress, anxiety, and depression. They believe the benefits of mindfulness are related to its ability to dial down the body's response to stress.

Much of the research on mindfulness has focused on two types of interventions, which you could do on your own or with others. Mindfulness-based stress reduction (MBSR) is a therapeutic intervention that involves weekly group classes and daily mindfulness exercises to practice at home, over an eight-week period. MBSR teaches people how to increase mindfulness through yoga and meditation. You could also see a therapist who practices mindfulness-based cognitive therapy (MBCT), a therapeutic intervention that combines elements of MBSR and cognitive behavioral therapy (CBT) to treat people with depression.

Outside of stress and depression, mindfulness has also been proven to improve immune function, an area where most women struggle especially during the menopausal transition (as discussed in chapter 2). Chronic stress can impair the body's immune system and make many other health problems worse. By lowering the stress response, mindfulness may have downstream effects throughout the body.

Vagal Nerve Work

Your vagus nerve is the longest nerve in the body, connecting your brain to your heart and your gut. It's part of your parasympathetic nervous system (the one that keeps you calm). Stimulating the vagus nerve helps you reduce anxiety by getting your body to move from a fight-or-flight response to a rest-and-digest response, slowing your heart rate and lowering blood pressure. Long-term, it can help with treatment-resistant depression, reduce inflammation, and increase your immune system's response. Here are myriad ways to stimulate your vagus nerve:

- **Deep breathing:** Inhale slowly through your nose, then exhale slowly through your mouth. You can try either the 4-7-8 breathing technique (breathe in for 4 seconds, hold for 7, and exhale for 8) or box breathing (breathe in for 4 seconds, hold for 4 seconds; breathe out for 4 seconds; hold for 4 seconds). Repeat if needed.
- **Meditation:** Focus on your breath and your surroundings in a quiet space for ten to fifteen minutes.
- **Humming or singing** for a few minutes can relax the vagus nerve.
- **Massage:** Gently massage the area behind your earlobe in small circles.
- **Cold facial stimulus:** Apply cold compresses to your face to increase vagal activity.
- **Nadi shodhana (alternate-nostril breathing):** Breathe gently through one nostril while closing the other with your finger. Swap.

Acupuncture

Acupuncture is a healing practice that originated in traditional Chinese medicine (TCM). It involves the insertion of very thin, sterile needles into specific points on the body, called acupoints, to stimulate the body's natural healing processes. The practice is based on the idea that the body has a flow of energy, or qi (pronounced "chee"), which travels through channels or pathways called meridians. When qi is blocked or imbalanced, it is believed to cause illness or discomfort. Acupuncture aims to restore balance to the flow of qi, thereby promoting physical and emotional well-being.

While the concept of qi is rooted in TCM, modern science suggests that acupuncture works through several biological mechanisms, including:

- Stimulation of the peripheral nervous system, sending signals to the brain and spinal cord, which can influence pain perception and promote healing
- Triggering the release of endorphins and other natural painkillers, reducing pain and promoting relaxation
- Possibly increasing blood flow to specific areas, promoting tissue repair and reducing inflammation
- Temporarily improving heart rate variability (HRV)
- Decreasing perception of stress
- Influencing immune system activity, enhancing the body's ability to fight infections and reduce inflammation
- Possibly regulating serotonin, dopamine, and other neurotransmitters, positively affecting mood and stress levels

Note: Consult your doctor before doing acupuncture if you have any bleeding disorders, cardiovascular disease, a pacemaker, active infections, seizure history, or diabetes.

Nature Exposure

Ah, the great outdoors. Fresh air, trees rustling, birds chirping . . . no wonder that nature exposure—spending time in natural environments like forests and parks, or near bodies of water—has significant benefits for both mental and physical health. It can help activate the parasympathetic nervous system and improve our mood, and it encourages mindfulness. It can reduce inflammation, too, and support a healthy microbiome by supporting the bidirectional nature of the gut and brain.

One activity that has been growing in popularity is forest bathing (shinrin-yoku), a Japanese practice of immersing oneself in a forest environment, which has demonstrated measurable reductions in stress hormones like cortisol and adrenaline (a.k.a. epinephrine). Spend time in a forest or wooded area, engaging your senses by noticing the sights, sounds, and smells. But you don't have to find a forest to get the benefits. Simple gardening and handling soil exposes you to beneficial microbes like *Mycobacterium vaccae*, which may improve mood and gut health. If you live in a city and don't have the outdoor space, walking outdoors will do the trick—just try to find a green space to combine the benefits of movement with nature exposure.

Holotropic Breathwork

You may be thinking, "Holo what?" But this promising new treatment, first coined by psychiatrist Stanislav Grof, who developed it in the 1970s, is a prolonged mindful breathwork to induce an altered state of consciousness. The practice is usually combined with evocative music in a special setting, done in groups led by a specially trained teacher.

Holotropic breathwork can help people process traumatic memories and experience emotional catharsis. It can also help them to become more self-aware, increase their self-esteem, and make them feel more connected to others. In addition, it can help reduce anxiety and depression: A meta-analysis published in *Scientific Reports* evaluated various breathwork techniques, including holotropic breathwork, and found that they may be effective in reducing stress and improving mental health.

Studies are ongoing, but researchers at Johns Hopkins University are investigating the efficacy of holotropic breathwork as a therapeutic intervention for veterans with PTSD, and their initial findings are promising, indicating that the practice can in fact help individuals better process traumatic experiences. (I have started integrating this in my own meditation and it has been a powerful experience.)

Note: This type of breathwork can bring up *intense* feelings. Because of this, it's not recommended for some people (e.g., those with heart disease, high blood pressure, or a history of seizures). Talk to your healthcare provider before practicing this type of breathing.

PEMF

PEMF, or pulsed electromagnetic field therapy, uses low-frequency electromagnetic waves to stimulate cells, tissues, and overall body function. It was first developed to heal bone fractures and improve circulation, and it has been shown to offer great relaxing and stress-lowering benefits as well. There are different types of devices, including full-body mats and portable devices, all of which can be bought online.

How does it work to reduce stress? It modulates the activity of the central nervous system, enhances neurotransmitter production, and promotes relaxation in individuals with stress. Studies have shown that PEMF therapy can improve relaxation by modulating brain-wave activity, promoting alpha waves and reducing beta waves (associated with stress and anxiety), while also reducing cortisol levels. Clinical studies also show an easing of anxiety and depression following PEMF treatments.

I love my mat and use it every day. If you want to try, start with two or three days per week for ten to fifteen minutes at a time. They range in price from a few hundred dollars to a couple thousand dollars, so do your research and get what fits your budget and priorities.

Note: Never use PEMF if you have implanted devices, like a pacemaker, cochlear implant, insulin pump, or other electronic devices.

Apollo Neuro

Sounds like the name of a space station, doesn't it? The Apollo Neuro is actually the first wearable system to improve heart rate variability, focus, and relaxation.

Neuro looks like a bracelet, but you can wear it on your wrist or on your ankle. The idea behind it is about our senses: Much like how music can relax us and touch can soothe us, vibration can have a similar effect. Originally designed for veterans with PTSD, the gadget uses vibration to reduce stress levels and get you out of the sympathetic into the parasympathetic system to improve heart rate variability. The gadget is still pretty new, but the company's informal studies show promising relief from stress and anxiety. The bracelet costs a few hundred dollars, but with daily wear, that can be worth every penny.

Neurofeedback

Neurofeedback is a therapeutic technique that provides real-time feedback, often through visual or auditory cues, to train individuals to regulate their brain activity and modulate their responses to stressors. Studies show there is a statistically significant improvement in symptoms in patients with

PTSD or generalized anxiety disorder (GAD), as well as significant improvement in subjective stress levels.

How does neurofeedback do this? It operates on the principle of neuroplasticity—the brain's ability to reorganize itself by forming new neural connections. After it measures real-time brain activity, the next step is training the brain with positive feedback or rewards. The training is not unlike training a dog to sit (really!). We like rewards, and this feedback gives it to us, leading to improved moods and reduction in the anxiety brought on by menopause.

Home devices run the gamut—from Muse to Mendi, Sens.AI, and NeurOptimal—but make sure you go to a healthcare professional who has certification and proper training. If you decide to use this strategy, find a medical professional who's certified through either the Biofeedback Certification International Alliance (BCIA) or Othmer Method Certification.

Changes to the brain typically happen slowly and over time. For that reason, it can take many sessions to achieve long-term changes in symptoms and brain functioning. As with all forms of exercise and therapy, it's best to do neurofeedback training regularly, usually two or three times a week. Costs vary, dependent on the device or the mental health provider's fees, but an average session costs between one hundred and two hundred dollars.

Note: Use neurofeedback with caution if you have preexisting neurological conditions, addiction, eating disorders, or psychiatric history.

Somatic Therapy

Also known as body-experiencing therapy, this is a practice that helps people with their anxiety and PTSD by teaching them to focus on bodily sensations with movements, gestures, postures, breath, and touch rather than relying on thought and emotion. Still with me?

It may sound woo-woo, but it is grounded in solid science. Amanda Baker, director of the Center for Anxiety and Traumatic Stress Disorders and a clinical psychologist in the Department of Psychiatry at Massachusetts General Hospital, calls it a "treatment focusing on the body and how emotions appear within the body. . . . Somatic therapies posit that our body holds and expresses experiences and emotions, and traumatic events or unresolved emotional issues can become 'trapped' inside." This requires a specialized therapist who can guide a patient through the exercises, and it's designed for PTSD.

Another similar technique, Somatic Experiencing (SE), is also a body-focused therapy designed to help individuals process and release stress and trauma. It was developed by Dr. Peter Levine and is based on the idea that trauma and chronic stress get "trapped" in the nervous system, leading to dysregulation and symptoms like anxiety, tension, and hypervigilance. SE helps reset the autonomic nervous system by allowing the body to gradually release stored stress energy. Studies are ongoing, but preliminary findings show positive effects of SE on PTSD-related symptoms. If you are struggling with PTSD or some form of trauma, I recommend you ask your provider or therapist about these two groundbreaking therapies.

You can try out a more basic form of SE anywhere, anytime. It's called grounding—a practice of making direct contact with the surface of the earth. The theory is that connecting to the earth's electrical charge offers mental health benefits. How to do it? It's easy.

1. Go outside—whether that's your backyard, a park, or the beach. The key is to be in physical touch with nature.
2. Either walk barefoot, put your hands directly on the ground, or touch a tree, or if you are by the beach, go for a dip in the water.
3. Try to get a sense of body awareness by focusing on what you feel. This should have a calming effect.

SE can also take the form of breathwork, specifically diaphragmatic breathing, also called belly breathing:

1. Lie on your back with one hand on your chest and the other on your stomach.
2. Inhale slowly through the nose, keeping your chest as still as possible (the hand on your belly should be the one moving).
3. Exhale slowly through pursed lips.

Both exercises can help you get into the present moment and get away from any anxious feelings.

MDMA-Assisted Therapy

An experimental but promising area of current research is the use of psychedelic therapies to help people overcome major traumatic experiences. According to one study, these psychedelics (both plant- and synthetic-based) can help trigger "non-ordinary states of consciousness characterized by profound alterations in perception, emotion, spiritual availability and cognition." Psychedelics that have been used to this effect are MDMA, ketamine, and more traditional psychedelic therapies, like psilocybin, LSD, and mescaline. For purposes of this book, I will keep my focus on MDMA, because it has the most research supporting it.

MDMA is a substance that supports social connection—that is, it's an empathogen, with stimulant effects. It also reduces the activity of the limbic system (a.k.a. lizard brain, the emotional center) in a manner that allows us to recall emotionally charged memories with much less emotional intensity than historically associated with revisiting these experiences. Studies have shown that MDMA downregulates the limbic system and increases communication between the amygdala and hippocampus, enabling people to revisit past traumatic experiences with less fear and emotional volatility. It has been shown to decrease feelings of fear and defensiveness while increasing feelings of well-being, sociability, and trust. This therapy is not currently FDA-approved; however, there are existing clinical trials that are ongoing and promising.

***

Remember Jessica? After talking to her, we developed a plan to reduce her stress and mitigate some of the unresolved trauma she had in her childhood. She tried meditation and yoga, and started measuring her vitals on her Oura Ring. She also tried vagal therapies and made sure she had twenty minutes of sun and fresh air in the backyard every day. After a month or so, she really started to notice a difference in her irritability and stress responses, so she has continued with these practices, working them into her everyday life.

We also put her on hormone replacement therapy, which is yet another tool to relieve menopausal stress-related issues. In fact, there is so much to discuss on the subject of HRT that the next chapter is devoted to just that topic.

Chapter Summary

1. Find stress-management solutions and commit to them; it is a practice.
2. Be open-minded to new strategies.
3. Be honest with yourself if your childhood stressors contribute to maladaptive patterns in adulthood.
4. Consider therapy if you need an objective person to speak with and work on your "stuff."

References for this chapter can be found on my website: cynthiathurlow.com/themenopausegut-references

Chapter 10

To HRT or Not to HRT

I didn't really think too much about hormone replacement therapy until I needed it. Even with all I know about the body, I was ill-prepared for that first GYN visit when I explained to my physician that my periods had gotten *so* heavy in perimenopause, at the age of forty-three. I'm not sure why she didn't take me seriously, until, during my pelvic exam, she realized how heavy my cycle really was.

"OMG, you are really bleeding heavily!" she said. It was the first day of my period, but still.

I was only offered a few options to address the heavy bleeding—including being put on oral contraceptives and getting a hysterectomy—but none were acceptable to me. I knew too much, and I knew that there were other ways to address my heavy cycle that did not involve synthetic hormones or surgery.

There was no discussion about how oral progesterone might have helped this relative hormonal imbalance that we commonly see in perimenopause, or any lifestyle-related changes that might have been helpful, just contraceptives or surgery. Needless to say, I declined all her suggestions and instead found a wonderful local midwife, who honored what I wanted to do (no synthetic hormones or surgical interventions, unless absolutely necessary). This experience emboldened me to start speaking up and out about perimenopause, because if a Hopkins-trained NP didn't know what to expect in perimenopause and beyond, I knew that my patients didn't stand a chance. Mind you, 2015 was a very different time than we are in now, when women are finding their voices and menopause advocacy is having an incredible moment.

And now after consulting so many of my clients navigating middlepause, I realize I was lucky that my doctor even suggested as much as she did. My story echoed those of so many other women who are entering this new time in their lives, awakening to the fact that we have been let down by our medical community for generations. And we still are, as there is a long-standing stigma attached to the aging process, as well as to perimenopause and menopause, and with it a certain loneliness and anxiety that women feel in a culture that is so dismissive of the real and consequential—often avoidable—changes to our body at this time. Luckily for you, there are finally reevaluations of previous studies, as well as more advocacy and research being done on women in perimenopause and menopause and how these changes affect the body, as you have been reading throughout this book. There are now more forward-thinking doctors, nurse practitioners, physician assistants, and other healthcare professionals and advocates who are championing HRT so women can stop feeling invisible and invalidated and start to feel empowered to speak up for themselves. We spend 30 to 40 percent of our lifetime in menopause, and we want those years to be vital and self-reliant. No one should have to suffer or feel guilty for looking for ways to relieve symptoms. We don't have to "just live with it."

We have a long way to go. Get this: Today, only 4 percent of all women of menopausal age are prescribed FDA-approved hormone therapy for perimenopause and menopause in the United States. But it wasn't always that low: HRT started in the 1960s, and by the nineties, many women were taking Premarin, which was the most widely used form of estrogen prescribed in the United States—up to 40 percent of women were taking it for some period of time. In 2002, however, all that changed.

The Damage of the Women's Health Initiative

Nothing slowed down the progress in menopausal health and HRT more than the publication of the Women's Health Initiative (WHI), a major study sponsored by the National Heart, Lung, and Blood Institute (NHLBI), in 2002. Conducted over 10 years, it had 68,000 participants ages 50 to 79, and its mission was to evaluate HRT as a prevention of cardiovascular disease and fractures due to osteoporosis, while monitoring for an increased risk of breast cancer, endometrial cancer, blood clots, and dementia.

Instead, the study left millions of women's lives forever changed in its wake. The results showed that breast cancer and heart attacks rose when taking HRT, an assertion that rocked the health community, and seemingly overnight, HRT was painted as a big bad villain that offered more risks than benefits. I was working as an NP for a large cardiology practice at the time, and I had countless female patients describing their experiences and symptoms of being forced off their HRT; it ran the spectrum from sore, achy joints to palpitations to frequent UTIs. These women were crying, pleading in my office to advocate for them, but my physician colleagues told me to "stay in my lane." The saddest part is this was entirely preventable.

Why? Following a subsequent reanalysis of the WHI trial, newer studies contradicted the trial's findings, mainly showing that HRT in younger women or in early-postmenopausal women had a "beneficial effect on the cardiovascular system, reducing coronary disease and all-cause mortality." All this showed that the study had been riddled with problems—in particular:

1. **The age and health of participants.** The average age was sixty-three, and it went all the way to seventy-nine, which meant participants were at higher risk for disease. Additionally, the women in these WHI studies were twelve to fifteen years past the onset of menopause. Thus, they were without their premenopausal levels of estrogen and progesterone long enough to bring about

changes in various bodily functions that are the precursors of disease or of undiagnosed disease.

The researchers also did not take the women's risk factors into account, such as obesity, prior history of smoking, or metabolic health issues like high blood pressure and diabetes. Simply put, this was not a healthy population to sample from.

2. **The types of hormones used.** The WHI was a multifaceted trial, including two double-blind, placebo-controlled, randomized trials of postmenopausal HRT. The first arm included oral conjugated equine estrogens (CEE) at 0.625 milligrams daily and oral medroxyprogesterone acetate (MPA) at 2.5 milligrams daily versus placebo. The second arm studied patients with prior hysterectomies and treated them only with 0.625 milligrams of oral CEE per day. These two trials studied the risks and benefits of the patients on HRT intervention compared with placebo groups.

    They used oral synthetic estrogen (CEE—Premarin, which comes from pregnant mare's urine) and synthetic progesterone (MPA), which raised the risk of heart disease, stroke, blood clots, breast cancer, and dementia. The combination of synthetic estrogen and progestins did show a modest increase in risk for breast cancer, but only after five years of continuous use. After twenty years, participants' risk for mortality matched that of the control group, further negating these effects. Hormones used were given at higher doses and different formulations than what is prescribed today.

One of the major problems with the interpretation and misunderstanding of this study was that it emphasized relative risk rather than absolute risk. (Absolute risk is the difference between two risks, like the number of people who got sick out of everyone, whereas relative risk is the *ratio* between two risks—how likely one group is to get sick compared with another.)

Bottom line: The findings of the CEE and MPA study should have been that no significant risks were found for cardiovascular disease, invasive breast cancer, stroke, or venous thromboembolism.

HRT is ideally initiated in perimenopause or early menopause—the sooner, the better. But WHI tested the effects of HRT ten years or more after menopause. We now know that *when* women start HRT is critical in defining the benefits and consequences of doing so. Unfortunately, the damage of the study was done, and we are still seeing the fearfulness of healthcare providers and women who are resistant to the idea of prescribing or using HRT, even though so much evidence shows its benefits *far* outweighing its risks. No alternatives provide the range of benefits offered by estrogen across multiple organ systems. HRT can provide effective relief for a wide variety of health conditions, potentially avoiding the need for multiple treatments for separate problems. But unfortunately the misinterpretation of this study negatively affected how women viewed HRT, and many clinicians did not feel comfortable prescribing it. This one big study drowned out all the other data that showed if you start HRT within ten years of menopause, it can reduce risks of coronary disease, osteoporosis, and dementia. The use of HRT dropped dramatically as everyone took the worst of the study to heart.

In 2022, the Menopause Society, the largest North American organization of providers who specialize in menopause, published the long-awaited "2022 Hormone Therapy Position Statement of the North American Menopause Society." In it, they state that hormone therapy remains the most effective treatment for vasomotor symptoms (VSM) and genitourinary syndrome of menopause (GSM), and that HRT has been shown to prevent bone loss and fracture. There were tons of clarifications, such as the importance of periodic reevaluation of a woman's benefit/risk profile with recommendations for appropriate dose, duration, family history, and so on in all decision-making, but the statement was sorely needed in the medical community. Finally, a public rebuke of the WHI study.

The tide is shifting. Much more education and effort are needed in order to influence prescribing practices and to ensure women are well informed. It will take healthcare providers and researchers many years to change the current thinking on HRT, and we have seen promising steps toward embracing it, thanks to many female voices out there doing the research and advocating for women. Until then, what you can do is arm yourself with the latest scientific information and decide what is best for you. This chapter is a great place to start!

The Case for HRT

The first place to start is to talk about how HRT can be beneficial for so many women. Although this book is focused on the microbiome, the benefits of HRT cannot be understated and might, in fact, be life-changing for you.

Helps Alleviate Most Menopausal Symptoms:

- 35 percent reduction in hip fractures and osteoporosis
- 35 percent decrease in new-onset diabetes
- 60 percent reduction in UTIs
- Improvement in insomnia
- Improvement in vaginal dryness
- Improved neurocognitive health
- Reduced night sweats and hot flashes
- Reduced risk of certain cancers, such as a 63 percent relative-risk reduction in colon cancer
- Promotes a healthy weight

Fixing your hormonal imbalance will lead to other great benefits.

Improves the Gut Microbiome

A study published in *Menopause* examined the microbiomes of postmenopausal women receiving HRT compared with those not undergoing therapy. The findings indicated that HRT recipients had a gut microbiome composition more similar to that of premenopausal women, suggesting that HRT may help maintain a premenopausal-like gut microbial environment. Although observational (meaning further research is needed), another study, highlighted in the journal *Maturitas*, discussed the estrogen–gut microbiome axis and the likely therapeutic implications of HRT on the gut microbiome.

Improves the Cardiovascular System

The number one killer of women is heart disease, and HRT can play a huge role in helping women reduce this risk. Estrogen helps maintain a healthy lining of blood vessels (endothelium), lowering the risk of plaque buildup. It also reduces the incidence of ischemic events (decreased blood supply). This leads to better vasodilatation (dilation of blood vessels), reduced blood pressure, increased blood flow, and improved cardiac performance.

Bottom line:

1. All the research suggests that women should initiate HRT either in perimenopause or within five years of transitioning into menopause to reduce the risk of side effects and disease. There's consensus about the "window of opportunity" being within the first ten years of menopause.
2. Every woman deserves to have a targeted discussion with their healthcare provider weighing the pros and cons of HRT, based on their personal medical history, genetics, family history, and lifestyle.
3. Not every woman has the obvious menopause symptoms (hot flashes, irritability), so women should read up on the silent symptoms as well as the benefits of HRT for brain, bone, and heart health.

Taking That Step

If you are thinking of HRT, talk to your healthcare provider (more on how to do that on page 196). Everyone is different, and something that's important to you may not be important to the next woman. Some women have hot flashes, some don't. Some suffer mood swings from hell, some don't. Some lose their libido, some don't. You know your body, and you'll need to weigh the risks and rewards. If there is a high risk in your family history for Alzheimer's, bone fractures, or any of the other things that we know estrogen is beneficial in reducing the risk of, that needs to be part of the discussion. If osteoporosis is a high risk factor in your family, improving bone health may be more important to you than if there is no family history of the disease.

The first thing your healthcare provider will need to do is to get your detailed history. There are some relevant aspects of your personal, family, or social history that are imperative to address:

1. Is there any personal or family history of breast, ovarian, or colorectal cancer? Obesity, diabetes, or poor metabolic health? Any history of miscarriages or gestational diabetes?
2. Any personal or family history of endometrial cancer? Risk factors for endometrial cancer include: Standard American Diet, eating ultraprocessed foods, obesity, sedentary lifestyle, history of diabetes or poor metabolic health.
3. Any personal or family history of deep vein thrombosis (blood clots in legs), recent surgery, or history of pulmonary embolus (blood clot in lungs)?
4. Any history of tobacco use? (Nicotine can age your ovaries prematurely and transition you into menopause earlier.)
5. Pre-HRT testing checklist: blood pressure, DXA scan, body composition evaluation with a bioimpedance scale to determine your fat-free mass to lean muscle tissue, breast health evaluation

via mammogram, pap smear. (See chapter 11 for more information.)

Common Types of HRT

This is where things get complicated. There are so many variations and combinations out there on the market that it can be really overwhelming, even for the most dedicated healthcare provider. But don't worry! I do my best to untangle this web of information here. But remember, it is best to talk to a licensed medical professional who can help you figure what is best for you and your individual needs.

First, there are many types of HRT, but let's focus mainly on replacing estrogen, progesterone, and testosterone. That's the easy part. Now comes the harder part: There are three main forms in which these replacement hormones are made:

Bioidentical hormones are derived from natural sources and have the same chemical structure as those naturally produced in the body. They are produced in the laboratory from plants (wild yams, cactus, or soy), but the structure and functions of these hormones are identical to that of the hormones made by the body.

Because they are "identical," they mimic the hormone more closely than a synthetic version. These are regulated by the FDA. Bioidentical estrogen is called estradiol; bioidentical progesterone is progesterone. These can be made by the pharmaceutical companies or compounded. Fun fact, there is currently no FDA-approved version of testosterone for women, so we either have to use one tenth of a male dose (AndroGel) or have it compounded. We hope there will be an FDA-approved testosterone in the future, but for now, we have these two options.

Synthetic hormones are artificially created and manufactured by pharmaceutical companies, and they're subject to strict FDA regulations. They come in tablets, patches, and gels. Progestins are the synthetic form of progesterone, and there are many versions of synthetic estrogen, including Premarin, the conjugated equine estrogen.

Compounding hormones are plant-derived bioidentical hormones that are made in a pharmacy (rather than a pharmaceutical company) and individualized for a particular person's needs. They come in capsules, troches, patches, creams, lozenges, and vaginal suppositories. Providers can tailor doses based on a woman's needs. Compounded bioidentical hormones are not FDA-approved (they do not require approval because they are not mass-produced), although the hormones obtained to make the compounded medications come from FDA-inspected and -approved facilities, and the pharmacists are regulated by US Pharmacopeia and the Code of Federal Regulations. Please note: Most FDA-approved HRT is covered by insurance, but compounded hormones rarely are. However, many compounding pharmacies can use payment from funds from your FSP (flex spending plan).

Current FDA-approved options:

Estrogen only

Alora patch (estradiol)
Cenestin pill (synthetic conjugated estrogens/SCEs)
Climara patch (estradiol)
Delestrogen shot (estradiol valerate)
Divigel gel (estradiol)
Elestrin gel (estradiol)
Enjuvia pill (SCE)
Esclim patch (estradiol)
Estrace pill or vaginal cream (estradiol)
Estraderm patch (estradiol)
Estrasorb skin cream/emulsion (estradiol)
Estring vaginal insert (estradiol)
EstroGel (estradiol)
Evamist transdermal spray (estradiol)
Femring vaginal ring (estradiol acetate)
Femtrace pill (estradiol acetate)
Imvexxy vaginal insert (estradiol)
Menest pill (esterified estrogen)

Menostar patch; only used to treat osteoporosis (estradiol)
Minivelle patch (estradiol)
Ogen pill or vaginal cream (estropipate)
Osphena pill (estrogen agonist/antagonist)
Premarin pill, vaginal cream, or injection (SCE)
Vagifem tablet (estradiol)
Vivelle patch (estradiol)
Vivelle-Dot patch (estradiol)

Note: Oral estrogen has more side effects because of a complex process related to metabolism in the liver. I personally like the patch because it is a "set it and forget it" option. You change it twice week, versus using creams and oral estrogen daily. However, oral estrogen can be a safe option for the right person.

Progesterone only
Prometrium pill (micronized progesterone that is immediate release)

Progestin only (synthetic)
Provera pill (medroxyprogesterone acetate)

Combination estrogen and progestin meds
Activella pill (estradiol/norethindrone acetate)
Angeliq pill (estradiol/drospirenone)
Climara Pro patch (estradiol/levonorgestrel)
CombiPatch (estradiol/norethindrone acetate)
Femhrt pill (ethinyl estradiol/norethindrone acetate)
Prefest pill (estradiol/norgestimate)
Prempro pill (conjugated estrogens/medroxyprogesterone)

Testosterone
Please note, there is no current FDA-approved testosterone option for women. Women can use either one tenth of the dose of AndroGel or compounded testosterone.

Common Misconceptions

Why HRT is *not* combined oral contraceptives (COCs)

I can't tell you how frequently patients or clients will excitedly share with me that they are finally on HRT . . . then they tell me what they were prescribed, and often it is, in fact, oral contraceptives. HRT and oral contraceptives are not one and the same. If you are prescribed COCs for contraception, then this is a different discussion, but many patients are told that they are prescribed HRT when in fact what they are prescribed is not HRT.

First, COCs are designed to suppress ovulation and prevent pregnancy, whereas HRT is designed to help control symptoms of perimenopause and menopause. The dosing of oral contraceptives is also much higher than that of HRT. So, definitely not the same.

Why progestin is *not* bioidentical to progesterone

My biggest issue is that we have better options than synthetic progestin. In specific circumstances, like using a progestin IUD, I think it can be a reasonable option for women, especially as they are transitioning from perimenopause into menopause, but oral micronized progesterone is superior in every aspect to progestin.

What HRT works for your symptoms

Why take progesterone: Low progesterone shows up as anxiety, depression, irritability, and insomnia; adding in oral progesterone can help. It can also be helpful for reducing heavy menstrual cycles, if you are still having your periods.

Why take estrogen: Estrogen helps alleviate hot flashes, insomnia, vaginal dryness, painful sex, changes in libido, low bone mass (osteopenia, osteoporosis), heart palpitations, dry skin, loss of collagen and elastin (causing wrinkles), brain fog, poor memory, and joint pain.

Why take testosterone: For better executive function, motivation, and support in building muscle, and to counteract changes in body composition and low libido.

Many women do best with all three medications, but bio-individuality rules, as we all experience middlepause differently. Not all women need to have their testosterone replaced; some simply continue making enough in menopause. I personally use all three: an estrogen patch (bioidentical, FDA-approved pharmaceutical), progesterone (bioidentical, compounded) because I prefer a sustained release formulation and it helps with sleep, and testosterone (bioidentical, compounded).

None of these therapies should be financially burdensome. For example, my estrogen patch is five dollars a month, so it's super inexpensive; my progesterone is a hundred dollars for ninety days, and so is my testosterone. Sixty-five dollars a month for HRT is well worth all the benefits I get from it (just ask my husband and kids!).

Common Questions

How long until you feel effects of HRT?

It depends on the person, and bio-individuality rules; typically, the longer you've been without hormones, the longer it may take to alleviate symptoms. It can be weeks up to a couple of months, but you will feel it working, in the form of reduced hot flashes and night sweats, as well as improved mood and sleep.

Possible side effects

While every woman is different, some may experience bloating, headaches, irritability, mood changes, fatigue, bleeding, breast tenderness or fullness, nausea, diarrhea, weight gain or weight-loss resistance, rash, itching, acne, or changes in libido. Some side effects are temporary, while others may be more persistent. Always discuss side effects or concerns with your provider.

How long are you on them?

This is symptom-dependent. Most of the research and experts now suggest that women should be able to remain on HRT for the rest of their lives.

WHY PELLETS ARE NEVER MY FIRST CHOICE OR RECOMMENDATION

A hormone pellet is a small implant that is placed in your hip or buttock that releases hormones into the bloodstream. It is approximately the size of a grain of rice. Once it is inserted, you cannot remove it, and whatever symptoms you experience, you are stuck with them for the duration of the pellet therapy, which tends to be three to six months. Now, this is why I don't like them:

- I have heard of some predatory practices. These are expensive and thus profitable. Some clinics may offer them without regard for the best interests of the patient.
- Some clinicians only take a weekend course on how to administer them and then start using them in their practices without much more experience. If you do decide to go with pellets, make sure you are in the hands of a very experienced clinician. There will likely be fewer side effects than with an individual who has less experience and is less knowledgeable. Their efficacy can be wildly unpredictable.
- It's more common to see bleeding than with other routes of administration.

Having That Conversation with Your Healthcare Provider

I know how important it is to feel like you have a voice in your own health, and with so many doctors and influencers creating a national conversation about menopause, I hope you feel emboldened to do so. Women can advocate for themselves by openly discussing and sharing their symptoms with healthcare providers, actively seeking information about treatment options, and being clear about their needs to ensure they receive appropriate care and support to manage their transition effectively.

Key ways to advocate for yourself during middlepause:

- **Educate yourself:** Learn about the different symptoms of perimenopause and menopause and the various treatment options available so you can have informed conversations with your healthcare team.
- **Open communication with your healthcare provider:** Be honest and detailed about your symptoms, including their severity and impact on your daily life. This is so important; there's no need to suffer in silence! Provide consistent feedback about what is working and what is not. Remember, this is a collaborative relationship, not a dictatorship.
- **Ask questions:** Don't hesitate to ask your provider about different treatment options, including HRT, lifestyle changes, supplements, and more.
- **Find a supportive healthcare provider:** Seek a licensed healthcare provider (physician, nurse practitioner, midwife, physician assistant, etc.) who is knowledgeable about middlepause and willing to listen to your concerns.

  Additionally, understand that it takes a village, including licensed healthcare providers like registered dieticians, physical therapists, pelvic floor experts with specialized training, and even mental health specialists (counselors, psychotherapists, cognitive-behavioral therapists, and mindfulness and meditation trainers).
- **Be assertive:** If you are not satisfied with your current treatment plan, advocate for adjustments or explore other options.
- **Talk to your employer:** If your middlepause symptoms are impacting your work performance, discuss reasonable accommodations like flexible hours or the option to work from home.
- **Join support groups:** Connecting with other women going through middlepause can provide valuable information, emotional support, and a sense of community.
- **Prioritize self-care:** Engage in healthy lifestyle practices like the right types of exercise, anti-inflammatory nutrition, digestive rest, stress management, and adequate sleep to manage symptoms effectively.

Important points to remember:

- **Don't be embarrassed to talk about perimenopause and menopause:** It's a natural part of life and should be discussed openly. I'm embarrassed to admit that I was super uncomfortable discussing this at first, until I realized that if we live long enough, perimenopause and menopause are natural ways our bodies age us out of our fertile years. It is OK!
- **Be prepared to advocate for yourself:** Know your symptoms and be ready to explain how they affect your life.
- **Seek support from loved ones:** Talk to your partner, friends, and family members about what you are experiencing.

Online Help

Once you've had that conversation about HRT with your internist, primary care physician, or GYN, they may still try to dissuade you from taking it. It's not their fault—information has been all but ignored in medical school, and progress to change that has been slow. But now there are alternatives popping up online, companies that have seen the need for women to find affordable and real healthcare for their menopausal needs. Every woman in perimenopause and menopause deserves access to high-quality care, and these telehealth companies can help fill in the blanks for GYNs, midwives, or PCPs who are less experienced or comfortable addressing HRT therapies. They range in cost, depending on your insurance coverage, but what I have found is reasonable (especially when it comes to your health!), and you can't beat the convenience factor. I would say these are great alternatives if you are looking for low-dose treatments for specific symptoms rather than a more comprehensive treatment, especially if you have a complicated medical history that may require an in-person evaluation and more rigorous follow-up. For full disclosure, I have not personally used these companies, and they may not all prescribe testosterone replacement.

Here is a breakdown of a few of them:

Alloy is an MD-only telehealth experience, so pricing is high, as you are paying for expertise. They have a host of diverse medications available outside of HRT options, including pills for gut health and skin/hair health.

Midi Health provides telemedicine by MDs and NPs; they are in all fifty states and have comprehensive insurance coverage for FDA-approved HRT as well as compounded options. I have no affiliation with any of these (although I have had Midi's chief medical officer, Dr. Kathleen Jordan, on my podcast), but I do think Midi seems the best in terms of accessibility and price. When I see a company charging $149 a month for an estrogen patch when it costs me five dollars a month through my local pharmacy, I get suspicious.

Winona is also a doctor-prescribed telehealth company available in thirty-three states, but it doesn't accept insurance, so its price tag is a little heftier than that of the other companies.

As with everything else, do your research. One way to figure out if you are a good candidate for HRT is testing. There is a lot out there, but the next chapter will help you make sense of all of it.

Chapter Summary

1. Work with a provider who will meet your expectations and needs.
2. Understand that HRT is just one piece of the middlepause puzzle. Lifestyle measures are equally important.
3. Research your HRT options.
4. Your middlepause experience is as unique as you are, so what worked for your BFF, sister, or colleague may be different from what works for you.
5. Know that you can always course correct.

References for this chapter can be found on my website: cynthiathurlow.com/themenopausegut-references

Chapter 11

Testing, Testing

I know the word *test* may give some people bad flashbacks to high school or college, but trust me, testing for our health is a good thing. If you can figure out a persistent problem, better manage your perimenopausal and menopausal symptoms, or detect something early on before it gets too serious, it can be life-changing. There are a zillion tests—way too many to cover in this book—but the following are what I think are the most common and beneficial from my many years of practice. I cover both conventional lab work as well as functional integrative medicine options because I believe both together can be very powerful tools for your overall health in middlepause—and beyond. Not all tests are necessary for everyone, but I will make the argument that baseline serum labs and stool testing are essential; the rest can be chosen based on symptoms, budget, and the simple desire for more information. Medicine is both an art and a science, and while everything that follows is backed by science, the testing itself—what to test, when, and how often—is a delicate art form.

Traditional Lab Work

These are very common tests that can be done by your primary care doctor or team—many of these can be part of your routine healthcare or prescribed on an as-needed basis.

Complete blood count (CBC) is one of the most common blood tests requested by clinicians—it is the best wide-range test that can pick up many health issues, such as infections, cancer, and other diseases, by evaluating the total numbers and characteristics of cell components in the blood, such as white blood cells (WBCs), red blood cells (RBCs), and platelets. It is also helpful to look for evidence of anemia with hemoglobin (Hgb) and hematocrit (Hct).

Comprehensive metabolic panel (CMP): This test measures your metabolism by looking at fourteen different levels such as electrolytes, liver enzymes, kidney function, proteins, glucose, and more. This gives you a quick, comprehensive perspective on these areas and allows you to determine if you need more testing. It can help detect the subtleties of diseases like insulin resistance, kidney or liver issues, and electrolyte abnormalities.

Thyroid panel: This panel measures a few things to help assess thyroid health, as it is common to see an underactive thyroid (hypothyroidism) in middle age. If you feel fatigued or have unexplained weight gain, this is one of the first tests I would do to ensure that your thyroid is functioning as it should be. An under-functioning and underactive thyroid is common in perimenopause and menopause. There are several types of thyroid blood tests, including TSH, which measures your thyroid secreting hormone; free T3, which measures your active thyroid hormone, triiodothyronine; free T4, which measures your inactive thyroid hormone, thyroxine; reverse T3, which if elevated shows signs of stress; and thyroid antibodies (anti-TPO and anti-thyroglobulin). Additionally, I like to look at thyroid cofactors, like iodine, iron, magnesium, selenium, zinc, copper, and sometimes B_{12} and folate, all of which are necessary for optimal thyroid health:

- **Iodine (I)** is an essential trace element that is a component of T4 and T3. Inadequate iodine intake can impair thyroid function and lead to goiters, cognitive-developmental disorders, and congenital abnormalities, collectively known as iodine-deficiency disorders.

- **Iron (Fe)** is essential to human health, as it brings oxygen to every part of the body. Iron deficiency adversely affects cognition, immune function, and thyroid health.
- **Magnesium (Mg)** has hundreds of functions in the body, but it plays a central role in thyroid disease. Mg is related to the stabilization of the structure of nucleic acids and seems also to be involved in DNA replication, transcription, and repair. I prefer testing red blood cell magnesium levels to standard serum magnesium for accuracy.
- **Selenium (Se)** is an important element in thyroid hormone biosynthesis and metabolism, and thyroid tissue has the highest Se concentration.
- **Zinc (Zn)** is essential for human health and plays a role in gene expression, cell division and growth, and a variety of enzymes involved in immune and reproductive functioning.
- **Copper (Cu)** maintains thyroid activity and lipid metabolism. Cu prevents T4 over-absorption and controls calcium levels.

Sex Hormones

These blood tests are helpful for a baseline assessment for a woman in perimenopause or menopause. For menstruating women, there are specific days we prefer testing estrogen, progesterone, FSH, and LH. If you are in menopause, these can be tested at any time.

- **Estradiol (E2)** is the predominant form of estrogen prior to menopause. Recall that it is wildly erratic before menopause, in the perimenopausal transition, so testing results can change day-to-day. Not all providers agree that it is necessary to test in perimenopause; however, I do like a baseline prior to initiating HRT. Note: You can also test estrone (E1) and estriol (E3).

- **Progesterone** shows lowered levels in early perimenopause, and this continues throughout the transition to menopause. Again, not all providers agree that it is necessary to test in perimenopause, as symptoms should guide therapy.
- **Testosterone** has two forms, "free" and "total," but free is the active form of the hormone, so that is what is typically tested. Not all women in menopause require testosterone replacement, but testosterone levels can be impacted by chronic stress as well. Not all providers test for this.
- **FSH (follicle-stimulating hormone):** This significantly rises during perimenopause, indicating the decline in a woman's ovarian reserve and the transition toward menopause. As the ovaries release fewer eggs, the pituitary gland releases more FSH in an attempt to stimulate them, leading to potentially irregular menstrual cycles and other perimenopausal symptoms.
- **LH (luteinizing hormone):** LH is a hormone secreted by the pituitary gland that triggers ovulation by signaling the ovaries to release a mature egg; in perimenopause it starts to rise as the ovaries release fewer eggs and estrogen starts to decline, causing the body to produce more LH in an attempt to stimulate ovulation and maintain estrogen levels.
- **Anti-Mullerian hormone (AMH)** can be tested for identifying ovarian reserve. An AMH test tells you the number of remaining eggs you have and whether your ovaries might be aging too quickly.

Other Hormone Blood Tests

Cortisol is your primary stress hormone, produced by the adrenal glands. A significant amount of cortisol dysregulation happens in middle age; I like to use both serum and urine- and saliva-based testing (discussed below). Cortisol follows a natural distribution throughout the day (according to circadian rhythm), and this can be monitored only through saliva or urine. So, a cortisol serum/blood test shows us total cortisol, while saliva tests show metabolized cortisol levels.

DHEA (dehydroepiandrosterone) is also produced in our adrenal glands; it is a precursor to both testosterone and estrogen. Chronic stress will deplete not only DHEA but also the rest of our sex hormones, so this becomes very important in perimenopause and beyond.

Lipids: Estrogen production is known to exert protective effects on lipid (fat) metabolism and on vascular health. As estrogen declines in perimenopause, there's a loss of those protective effects, leading to a higher risk of cardiovascular disease and atherosclerotic cardiovascular disease (ASCVD), which is the number one killer of women. Estrogen also changes our lipid profile, including a rise in LDL cholesterol and triglycerides with a concomitant decrease in HDL levels. So lipids and metabolic health lab tests can be very important in measuring our middlepause health.

In addition to a traditional lipid panel (total cholesterol, LDL, HDL, and triglycerides), I always like to monitor apolipoprotein B (ApoB) and lipoprotein(a), or Lp(a). Lp(a) is a specific lipid in the blood that's similar in structure to LDL but with an extra protein, and high levels of it can increase the risk of heart disease and stroke. These structural differences make Lp(a) seven to eight times more atherogenic than LDL. And Elevated Lp(a) is indicative of oxidative stress and inflammation within the lining of our blood vessels. One of the most interesting aspects of this lipid is that its level is determined by genetics in more than 90 percent of cases, with lifestyle habits having very little influence. So if your Lp(a) levels are low, you may never need to test again! Amazing, right? Apo B is the main protein found in LDL cholesterol, and it tends to increase in the menopausal transition and can be included as part of a comprehensive lipid panel to assess cardiovascular risk as accurately as possible.

Homocysteine levels are worth checking, too, as elevated levels are linked to higher levels of lipids, especially LDL cholesterol and triglycerides, so it can be another inflammatory marker. With shifts in estrogen, you can see a rise in homocysteine. If deficient in key B vitamins, like B_6, B_{12}, and folate, you may also see higher homocysteine levels. Finally, when I see a high ApoB and Lp(a) in a client, I'll order a Boston Heart Cholesterol Balance test, a nontraditional lab test that measures circulating plasma cholesterol, which can indicate an LDL-C lowering response to treatments (e.g., statins or ezetimibe). This test helps healthcare providers offer the best plan of action to their clients. This test is particularly helpful when I want to look a bit more deeply at baseline abnormal lipid levels, specifically ApoB and Lp(a), to determine what medication is most appropriate to use in addition to lifestyle measures.

Metabolic Health Markers

The following tests can be crucial in helping determine your metabolic health. As you know by now, menopause may bring with it an increased risk of developing metabolic syndrome, including more abdominal fat and worsening fasting insulin and blood glucose levels. This association may be due to loss of estrogen, which helps with insulin sensitivity, or it may be a more indirect result of the redistribution of body fat that can occur as estrogen levels decline. Fasting insulin and blood glucose levels are important markers of metabolic health, alongside lipid levels, triglycerides, blood pressure, and waist circumference. But regularly monitoring blood glucose and insulin levels can help middle-aged women fine-tune their lifestyle habits to support healthy fasting biomarkers, which will help decrease the risk of chronic health issues that accompany poor metabolic health and allow for early detection of insulin resistance or diabetes risk. Here are the various tests:

- **Fasting insulin** is typically the first lab that will shift with worsening metabolic function, way before the A1C or fasting glucose.
- **Hemoglobin A1C** is a ninety-day marker of glucose control; it's common to see a loss of insulin sensitivity as a woman progresses from perimenopause into menopause.
- **Hs-CRP**, or high-sensitivity C-reactive protein, is a more sensitive marker of inflammation; this typically rises in middlepause in the setting of declining estrogen.

- **ESR (erythrocyte sedimentation rate)** is less specific than hs-CRP, but it can show elevated levels with systemic (body-wide) inflammation.
- **Uric acid** is a marker for not only metabolic health but also inflammation. It is most commonly associated with accumulation in joints, or gout, but it can be a marker for insulin dysregulation as well.

Anemia Markers

While anemia is often associated with menstruating women due to the blood loss, iron-deficiency anemia can still occur in perimenopausal women. An iron deficiency adversely affects cognitive development and immune function. Vegetarians also have a higher risk for developing low iron stores, iron depletion, and associated iron-deficiency anemia, compared with nonvegetarians.

Anemia markers can provide information on iron levels as well as iron storage and can help a patient understand if they need to adjust their dietary intake accordingly. Iron levels tend to increase as women get closer to menopause and in postmenopause, as that monthly blood loss is no longer occurring.

Additionally, women using hormone replacement therapy to address perimenopausal or menopausal symptoms may experience lower iron levels, making monitoring anemia panels an important piece of data in an integrative approach to supporting these women. Adequate iron storage is important for maintaining good energy levels, as iron plays physiological roles in oxygen transport as well as energy production in the mitochondria. Here are the tests for anemia:

- **Iron** is essential to human health, as it participates in oxidation-reduction reactions and plays a role in oxygen transport in the body. Iron deficiency adversely affects cognition and immune function.
- **Ferritin** is the lab that identifies the actual amount of iron that is bioavailable, or stored in the body.

- **Transferrin saturation** is a blood test that measures the percentage of iron bound to transferrin in the blood. (Transferrin transports iron into the blood.)
- **TIBC (total iron-binding capacity)** measures how well your body carries iron throughout your body.

Other Labs That Measure Your Health

Vitamin D_3 (25-hydroxyvitamin D): Monitoring vitamin D levels during menopause is crucial. Declining estrogen levels can significantly increase the risk of vitamin D deficiency, which is strongly linked to decreased bone mineral density, leading to a higher risk of osteoporosis and fractures. Therefore, maintaining adequate vitamin D levels is vital for bone health in postmenopausal women. It has been shown that during menopause, women may be particularly susceptible to the consequences of vitamin D deficiency, because a decrease in bone mineral density and lean mass, as well as an increase in fat mass, occurs in this period of life as a result of the decrease in estrogen levels. Vitamin D is also a hormone precursor that plays a key role in immune function and mood, and deficiencies can be a factor in autoimmune disease and certain cancers.

Functional/integrative testing: In addition to conventional testing, there are functional tests that can prove invaluable in measuring our health. What's the difference? While conventional medical testing focuses on one area of the body, functional labs tend to test the body as a functioning unit. Unfortunately, because they aren't considered medically necessary by traditional healthcare companies, these are generally out-of-pocket expenses, so they may not be accessible for everyone. (For example, some companies won't send testing kits to New York state.) You should go to an experienced functional medical provider who is well-read on these tests and proficient in evaluating them.

Micronutrient testing (MN): During perimenopause, a woman's nutritional and nutrient needs change as her physiology changes. Micronutrients such as calcium, B vitamins, zinc, magnesium, and iron are essential for the hormone fluctuations and accompanying shifts in insulin sensitivity that are happening at this time. Vitamin C may be helpful for improving symptoms of cognitive decline that can occur with perimenopause. Calcium and vitamin D are essential to support bone health, an important issue as bone density starts to decrease with declining estrogen levels. Vitamin K, selenium, and beta-carotene have also been linked with better bone mineral density in postmenopausal women, so optimizing intake of these nutrients, as guided by testing, can be part of a proactive plan during perimenopause. The SpectraCell Micronutrient Test, discussed in the next section, can help identify vitamin or mineral deficiencies that may be exacerbating symptoms of hormone decline and can help guide personalized nutritional and supplement interventions to improve the quality of life for women in middlepause.

Who benefits from these tests? They can be helpful in menopausal individuals with mood disorders, poor metabolic health, fatigue, weight-loss resistance, malnutrition, malabsorption, cognitive decline, and trauma and healing. The tests can help guide recommendations around the need for methylation support, toxin exposures, mitochondrial dysfunction, fatty acid imbalances, and oxidative stress. You can request these tests from a functional or integrative practitioner.

Testing Options for Micronutrients

1. SpectraCell Micronutrient Test (cost: around $450)

This test is a comprehensive analysis tool that examines thirty-three essential vitamins, minerals, and other nutrients to pinpoint potential deficiencies and assess functional status. Micronutrients, including vitamins and minerals, are vital for maintaining normal metabolism, growth, and overall physical well-being. The Micronutrient Test assesses an individual's level of the following vitamins, minerals, and nutrients:

Vitamins

- Vitamin A
- Vitamin B_1
- Vitamin B_2
- Vitamin B_3
- Vitamin B_6
- Vitamin B_{12}
- Biotin
- Folate
- Pantothenate
- Vitamin C
- Vitamin D_3
- Vitamin K_2

Minerals

- Calcium
- Magnesium
- Manganese
- Zinc
- Copper

Amino Acids

- Asparagine
- Glutamine
- Serine

Fatty Acids

- Oleic acid

Antioxidants

- Alpha-lipoic acid
- Coenzyme Q10
- Cysteine
- Glutathione

- Selenium
- Vitamin E

Carbohydrate Metabolism

- Chromium
- Fructose sensitivity
- Glucose-insulin metabolism

Metabolites

- Choline
- Inositol
- Carnitine

2. The NutrEval panel by Genova Diagnostics (cost: around $439)

This is a comprehensive nutritional evaluation that identifies more than 125 specific biomarkers like vitamins, minerals, antioxidants, organic acids, amino acids, essential fatty acids, oxidative stress, and other elemental markers to help diagnose many chronic health issues.

Antioxidants help prevent cellular damage. The panel tests for necessary antioxidants that our bodies make as well as those that our bodies do not make and have to be consumed through our diets.

B vitamins are cofactors for enzymes and are essential to fundamental metabolic processes. Dietary sources are essential for the body to manufacture B vitamins; the panel tests for B_1 (thiamine), B_2 (riboflavin), B_3 (niacin), B_6 (pyroxidine), B_7 (biotin), B_9 (folic acid), and B_{12} (cobalamin).

Minerals play a key role as cofactors for a wide variety of enzymatic processes. Testing includes manganese, molybdenum, magnesium, and zinc.

Essential fatty acids are not made by the body but are required for optimal functioning of a variety of physiological processes. They must be obtained through diet to avoid deficiencies.

Digestive absorption is assessed, and recommendations are made in two categories to optimize digestion and absorption of macronutrients and micronutrients: pancreatic enzyme support and probiotic supplementation.

Amino acids are building blocks of protein, important for structural support, neurotransmitter and hormone synthesis, energy production, and detoxification. Testing for amino acid levels and dietary peptide-related markers provides insight into protein intake and breakdown.

Comprehensive Stool Testing

Stool testing is a must in my practice. These tests can uncover digestive issues of all types, which could be latent infections in the stomach or small or large intestine, imbalances in the microbiome, and so on. Evaluating the health of the gut microbiome is an important component of any plan to support optimal hormone health during perimenopause. The sex hormones and the gut microbiome influence each other, so a period of hormonal changes is likely to impact the makeup of the gut microbiota, which can in turn influence other hormone systems, digestive function, and other physiological roles (as discussed at length in chapters 1 and 4). As estrogen levels can fluctuate quite a bit in perimenopause and menopause, the relationship between estrogen and the gut microbiome can be an important lab assessment to help with patient results. A comprehensive digestive stool analysis can assess for aforementioned biomarkers such as beta-glucuronidase, evaluate for dysbiosis, and help identify if gut support is needed for optimal digestion and immune function.

There are many stool-testing options, but the following are the three companies that I use with the greatest frequency. These are not at-home tests; any of them will have to be ordered through and evaluated by a licensed healthcare provider.

1. GI360 Profile (cost: about $500)

The GI360 stool test, put out by Doctor's Data, uses, according to their website, a "gut microbiota DNA analysis tool that identifies and characterizes the abundance and diversity of more than 45 targeted analytes that peer-reviewed research has shown to contribute to dysbiosis and other chronic disease states." It can identify the presence of pathogenic viruses, bacteria, and parasites, so it is useful for GI symptoms, inflammation, joint pain, autoimmunity, food sensitivities, chronic or acute diarrhea, abdominal pain, and nutritional deficiencies.

2. GI-MAP test (cost: $350+)

This microbiome-focused stool test, which uses a quantitative polymerase chain reaction (qPCR) technology, is unique to the industry and captures low-level microorganisms. It screens for more than fifty bacterial pathogens, viruses, worms, parasites, various yeast types, *H. pylori*, and virulence factors that can disturb normal microbial balance and cause illness. Additionally, biomarkers related to inflammation, digestion, and immune function are included. Results of this test can be used to improve intestinal permeability and microbial diversity, which, as we know, can be impaired in perimenopause and menopause.

3. Genova GI Effects Stool Profile (cost: $439)

This test provides a broad overview of markers for inflammation, digestion and absorption, and the microbiome. It focuses on three key functions of gut health, including digestion, inflammation, and gut microbiome, and it also looks at five key areas of GI function: maldigestion, inflammation, dysbiosis, metabolite imbalances, and infection.

Food-Sensitivity Testing

Many women come to me with food-sensitivity issues. While food-sensitivity testing is controversial, as there is not enough research to back it up, I can say that in my clinical experience, I have seen patients suffer time and time again with foods they just can't seem to tolerate, and testing can help. I usually start with a simple elimination diet (like Whole30) for thirty days to reduce or eliminate foods your body may not be able to tolerate. Whole30 removes gluten, dairy, grains, soy, alcohol, and sugar, and then after thirty days, we reintroduce the foods gradually. The patient also keeps a food journal to monitor any and all symptoms. If this helps, then we can stop here and just monitor. If symptoms persist or the patient requests food-sensitivity testing, then we proceed with testing that can help identify which foods potentially trigger inflammation and symptoms. Results can be used to develop a personalized elimination diet to support gut healing.

Two tests that I use:

Genova's Food Sensitivity (cost: $429): This uses finger stick, and it can test food and environmental sensitivities. There are also other options, including the IgG Food Antibody test ($125).

Mediator Release Test (MRT) (cost: around $300): This test is taken by drawing blood.

I offer food-sensitivity testing with my patients if they have the following signs:

- Irritable bowel syndrome (IBS)
- Major depressive disorder
- Migraine headaches
- Skin rashes such as eczema
- Joint aches
- Autoimmune disease
- Crohn's disease
- Obesity or weight-loss resistance

Food-Allergy Testing

A food allergy is different from a sensitivity; this is a severe immune response to a food, which is often caused by increased production of an antibody called immunoglobulin E (IgE). Symptoms occur within two hours and may include hives, tongue swelling, difficulty breathing or swallowing, and dizziness. Food allergies can be life-threatening. Food sensitivities, on the other hand, are believed to be an immune reaction driven by antibodies such as immunoglobulin G (IgG), immunoglobulin M (IgM), and immunoglobulin A (IgA), along with other cell-mediated reactions in your body in response to specific foods or groups of foods. Symptoms may include digestive distress (gas, diarrhea, abdominal pain), joint pain, brain fog, and migraine. These symptoms may be subtle or may not happen right away. Food sensitivities are not life-threatening.

Here are some differences between IgE-mediated allergic reactions and IgG-mediated food sensitivities:

IgE-Mediated Allergies (foods, molds, inhalants)

- Immediate onset (minutes to hours)
- Circulating half-life of one to two days
- Permanent allergies
- Mast cell activation
- Stimulates histamine release
- Hives, stuffy or itchy nose, sneezing, itchy or teary eyes, vomiting, stomach cramps or diarrhea, angioedema or swelling, shortness of breath or wheezing, anaphylaxis

IgG-Mediated Sensitivities (foods, spices, vegetarian foods)

- Delayed onset (hours to days)
- Circulating half-life of twenty-two to ninety-six days
- Temporary sensitivities
- Does not stimulate histamine release

- Gastrointestinal symptoms, headaches, joint pain, skin rashes, fatigue, behavioral problems, other vague symptoms

The role of IgG food antibody testing is still being researched; however, studies have shown the benefits of testing in certain conditions.

Additional Types of Testing: Hormone Testing

1. Precision Analytical DUTCH (cost: $350+)

The DUTCH (dried urine test for comprehensive hormones) test specializes in the assessment of hormone health. It's a relatively new technology that provides additional information in hormone metabolite testing. I like this test for looking at the distribution of cortisol secretion throughout the day and looking at estrogen metabolism (how it is broken down). There are two options available, DUTCH Plus and DUTCH Complete, but I prefer the former since it provides both urinary metabolites and saliva data.

The DUTCH Plus incorporates both urine and saliva samples to measure the cortisol awakening response (CAR), alongside the standard sex and adrenal hormone assessments. This test is particularly valuable for understanding the body's response to stress upon waking, which can be crucial for patients dealing with anxiety, depression, or chronic stress conditions. The results concerning the circadian distribution of cortisol throughout the day are very insightful, along with information around estrogen detoxification patterns. This test is helpful, but not necessary.

2. ZRT Laboratory (cost: $380)

I do not use this lab as often as Precision Analytical, but it can be helpful in specific circumstances. Comprehensive Female Profile II uses saliva and small samples of blood, called a blood spot. This test helps provide insights into sex hormones and thyroid and adrenal health markers.

Now that you have had a good primer on testing, let's check out supplements that may help improve your test results and get you on the road to better health.

Chapter Summary

1. Testing can help determine or rule out serious health problems early or help maintain your health by measuring macro- and micronutrients.
2. Find a health provider who understands your needs and will work with you on what testing is best for your health history.
3. Do research to see what is available to you (or your health provider).

References for this chapter can be found on my website: cynthiathurlow.com/themenopausegut-references

Chapter 12

An Extra Dose of Support

I view supplements as precisely that—supplemental. It is so easy in our "ready-made" culture to just take a supplement and not actually change our diet, but there is no magic pill that will fix things for us without changing our nutrition and lifestyle patterns. Supplements should be something we reach for only if there is an issue with getting what we need from food. What I have included in this chapter are supplements I find most effective for women at this stage of life for a variety of benefits: improved digestion, generalized gut support, polyphenols, stronger bones, and better sleep, stress resilience, and immunity. This is not an exhaustive list because, quite frankly, there are just so many supplements out there, and it is also dependent on every woman's individual needs. So, as always, consult your healthcare provider, who should review your health history and nutritional habits and conduct any lab work before recommending supplements. Also, please consult your provider if there are any possible contradictions. For example, these should not be taken if pregnant, trying to conceive, or breastfeeding, or if you have liver or renal issues.

Note: Although supplements, both the products themselves and the ingredients, are regulated by the FDA, they're not generally subject to the same testing and regulations as medications. And, according to the FDA, while there are laws for marketing companies and manufacturers to "evaluate both the safety and labeling" to ensure that they meet the requirements of the Federal Food, Drug and Cosmetic Act and protect consumers, it is important to carefully source supplements from reputable brands and watch out for those that are not FDA-approved. I hope to make all of what is out there easier to choose by providing some trusted and high-quality options for you in the Resources section. But remember, always talk to your health provider before taking anything.

The Gut

Digestive Supports

Because we produce fewer digestive enzymes as we get older, a lot of women have issues with bloating, indigestion, or reflux. The first thing I like to do is to recommend an elimination diet and then consider food sensitivity for persistent issues. I frequently recommend digestive supports, and I find these really effective.

A word of caution: Digestive supplements can be helpful, but for persistent symptoms, it is always best to be evaluated by either your internist, primary care provider, or a specialist to make sure you don't have any significant issues provoking symptoms that require further evaluation.

Digestive bitters are typically herbs with a bitter taste and have been used for centuries in many cultures, including traditional Chinese medicine and Ayurvedic medicine, to help support and maintain healthy digestion. These include burdock root, dandelion, schisandra, chamomile, gentian, ginger, and artichoke leaf. Even bitter greens (arugula, radicchio), citrus (think warm lemon water), and polyphenol-rich plant compounds found in bitter tea and coffee are all helpful for supporting our digestive system.

All bitters help stimulate our digestive systems, which includes secretion of saliva, hydrochloric acid (HCl), and bile; this can be hugely helpful in supporting a healthy digestive process. Bitters also stimulate the cascade of peristalsis.

I recommend these to patients who want overall digestive support, and to those who experience bloating, gas, low stomach acid (hydrochloric acid, or HCl) symptoms, gallbladder issues, or problems with protein or fat absorption.

Recommended dose: Depends on the product, can use with meals

Digestive enzymes (DE) are proteins produced and secreted by the gastrointestinal system that help break down the foods you eat so you can use them as energy. Your body produces many different types of enzymes to help digest carbohydrates, proteins, and fats. It is not uncommon to see issues surrounding gallbladder health, like an inability to break down and assimilate fats, or inflammation or infections, at this stage of life.

Some research suggests that digestive enzymes may allow for better absorption of nutrients for those with celiac or other autoimmune disorders; they also may help those with lactose sensitivity. I will recommend these to patients with bloating, gas, and low-HCl symptoms, possibly along with an elimination diet while we are waiting on testing results. Some important enzymes include the following (most supplements include many of these in some combination):

- **Amylase:** Breaks down complex carbs in starchy foods like bread, sweet potatoes, and beans into simple sugars
- **Lactase:** Breaks down lactose, the sugar in milk and cheese
- **Protease:** Breaks down proteins in foods like eggs, meat, and fish into amino acids
- **Lipase:** Breaks down fats from foods like nuts, oils, and butter into fatty acids
- **DE:** Can also be helpful after an elimination diet or food-sensitivity testing to help evaluate gas, bloating, loose stools or diarrhea, constipation, and so on

Recommended dose: Depends on the product

TUDCA (tauroursodeoxycholic acid) is one of my favorite supplements, as it increases bile flow. A naturally occurring bile acid, it has been used for millennia in Chinese medicine on liver and gallbladder conditions, such as cholestasis, the impairment of bile flow from the liver. After many years of fats being vilified, I find that many patients require some degree of bile support, as they have been either avoiding healthy fats or consuming the adulterated versions (rancidified seed oils, as one example). The avoidance of fats contributes to viscous bile that can make it harder for our gallbladder to function. When the bile is too thick, it can lead to blockages, infections, and symptoms like right upper quadrant pain (RUQ), nausea, and vomiting. This phenomenon is sometimes referred to as gallbladder sludge (ew).

What is bile? It's a yellowish-green digestive fluid produced by the liver designed to help break down and emulsify fats. It's sort of like how dishwashing soap helps to break down grease when you're washing dishes. If your body cannot break down and emulsify fats properly, it can lead to dysbiosis and fat malabsorption (which includes our fat-soluble vitamins A, D, E, and K), and it can contribute to a leaky gut. Not only does the research show that individuals who supplement with TUDCA experience an increase in bile, but the *composition* of their bile also changes, containing higher amounts of compounds that positively assist digestion. It also has cytoprotective properties, meaning it helps protect cells from damage caused by stress, including oxidative stress, which can be exacerbated during menopause due to hormonal fluctuations. In addition, TUDCA can reduce inflammation, and it has been shown in preclinical models to improve insulin sensitivity. Reducing inflammation, in particular, can help further support our gut microbiome in perimenopause and beyond.

Recommended dose: 250–1,500 mg daily; higher doses may cause diarrhea. For best results, take it in cycles: 30 days on, 30 days off.

Note: Do not use if you are pregnant or nursing. If you have any chronic health conditions, please discuss with your healthcare team first, as it has the potential to interact with other medications.

Gut Support

This is another shelf space where there is so much to choose from, but the following are ones that I have found most helpful for my patients.

Fiber is crucial to our health during middlepause to combat the changes to our gut microbiome at this stage. Consuming fiber is an excellent way to improve the diversity of our gut microbiota, as it helps feed our colonocytes. It can also help with blood sugar stabilization, weight management, healthy stools, and more. I prefer my patients to get enough fiber—about twenty-five grams daily—from food, but if they can't, supplementation is OK. You can track your fiber intake with something like the Cronometer app.

If you opt for a fiber supplement, go low and slow with dosing to avoid digestive bloating, gas, or constipation. A combination of vegetables, low-glycemic fruits, and a bit of additional supplementation seems to work best.

Immunoglobulin G (IgG) supports immune function, especially for those individuals who need additional help but need a dairy-free source. It helps maintain a healthy intestinal immune system by binding to microbes and toxins in the gut. It can also help enhance mucosal immunity, maintain microbial balance, and support GI barrier health and integrity.

I like to use these if results of stool testing suggest a low immune function in the digestive system along with symptoms and recent illness or antibiotic use. I also find that supplements like colostrum tend to be less well tolerated because so many women are sensitive to cow milk.

Recommended dose: Depends on individual product; avoid if you have a beef allergy

L-glutamine is an amino acid that is used as food by the cells that line the gut. It can be found in beef, eggs, milk, and other animal products, and it is also a good supplement to add, as it is integral for both immune health and our microbiome. It helps repair and maintain the gut lining. It is a primary fuel source for enterocytes (gut cells), and it helps to seal the tight junction proteins, like occludin and zonulin, in the gut and keep the gut lining in a pristine and healthy state. It helps support a healthy microbiome in the gut and helps to reduce inflammation. Use of L-glutamine can even support nutrient absorption in the small intestine and help promote regular bowel movements.

Research shows that our immune cells depend on L-glutamine to survive, multiply, function, and ultimately defend our body against pathogens. Specifically, it boosts the immune system by supporting the production of white blood cells. One study even showed that L-glutamine supplementation reduced the rate of hospital-acquired infections and reduced the length of stay in the hospital. Research has also shown it can reduce pro-inflammatory cytokine production, making it a great potential therapeutic for a host of inflammatory conditions. If that is not enough, L-glutamine has also been shown to aid in the production of serotonin, one of our neurotransmitters that, in addition to regulating mood, influence appetite signals. L-glutamine also promotes healthy weight loss by helping to improve insulin sensitivity.

Recommended dose: 4–8 mg daily

Nitric oxide (NO) is a molecule that is naturally produced in our bodies. It has specific effects on the dilation of blood vessels, the release of hormones, and communication between nerve cells (neurons). Our levels of nitric oxide drop in menopause, along with estrogen levels, impacting the health of our hearts, brains, metabolism, and circulation.

However, lifestyle choices, HRT, and targeted supplements can help restore NO levels and support overall well-being.

Signs of low NO include cognitive decline, high blood pressure, insulin resistance, weight gain, and poor exercise recovery (note, these are all aligned with changes that we see with women navigating perimenopause and menopause, too!).

Recommended dose: Varies

Polyphenols are considered to be one of the most important metabolites produced by plants and have a wide array of health benefits, including anti-inflammatory, antibacterial, antioxidant, and even neuroprotective effects. Most are not absorbed along our stomach or small intestine, but rather are transformed into active compounds in the large intestine courtesy of our gut bacteria. Even with diligence in terms of diet, I do appreciate the added benefits of supplementation.

There is additional research surrounding the use of (general) polyphenol supplementation in menopause and benefits to mental health. A study from 2021 in *Frontiers in Psychiatry* suggested that supplementation with polyphenols was effective at reducing depression. Polyphenols are noted to have potent anti-inflammatory properties that may positively impact depression and anxiety symptoms. Given the prevalence of mood disorders reported in middle-aged women—33.5 percent and 54.2 percent of women aged forty-five to seventy years old are estimated to have depression and anxiety, respectively—the value of supplemental support along with other lifestyle measures and HRT is undeniable.

One of my favorite polyphenols is *Akkermansia mucinophilia*, which is also a keystone bacterium. It helps with endogenous GLP-1 (glucagon-like peptide) production and satiety, as well as production of short-chain fatty acids, and it helps with mucus production in the lining of the small intestine. There is also emerging research showing that akkermansia is a promising strategy for treatment of poor metabolic health issues, which are increasingly common in the menopausal transition.

Recommended dose: Varies

Urolithin A is one of the most exciting developments in mitochondrial health. It is a postbiotic compound that helps clean out damaged mitochondria and promote the growth of healthy new ones. It is also beneficial for reducing inflammation. If you happen to be someone who has a healthy gut microbiome (lucky you), your gut bacteria can convert polyphenols from foods (like pomegranates, berries, and nuts) into postbiotics and metabolites like urolithin A. But only about 30 to 40 percent of people have the right gut bacteria to create meaningful amounts, and I find that most, if not all, of my female patients have a microbiome that is consistent with dysbiosis and requires a bit of support and assistance to flourish at this stage of life. Think of it as taking out the cellular trash—you need to clear out the old to make room for the new. Urolithin A helps with energy, muscle recovery, and mitochondrial health in older adults, and it may be a promising approach to counteracting age-associated muscle decline.

Recommended dose: 1,000 mg daily

Bones

Many supplements support healthy bones, and by no means is this an exclusive list—just the heavy hitters. Nearly every female patient needs vitamin D (especially if they live north of Atlanta) and magnesium supplementation. I also like collagen peptides, not only for bone support but also for hair, skin, and nails, and creatine monohydrate is a foundational, all-around supplement.

Collagen peptides help stimulate bone-building cells and improve bone density. Research suggests that it may also help prevent bone loss, particularly in menopausal women, through mechanisms like stimulating osteoblast activity and improving bone matrix quality. Research has also shown that regular intake of specific collagen peptides can lead to measurable increases in bone density in areas like the spine and femoral neck, indicating a potential benefit for managing osteoporosis.

Recommended dose: 5–15 g daily

Creatine monohydrate is one of the most heavily researched supplements on the market. It has become very popular because it has been shown to have the potential to influence bone biology, with or without resistance training. By increasing the activity of osteoblasts (cells involved in bone formation), creatine can reduce bone resorption (loss), and when combined with resistance training, it can increase the muscle-to-bone interaction. According to creatine researcher and expert Dr. Darren Candow, creatine monohydrate could supplement exercise in the management of osteosarcopenia (loss of muscle and bone with aging).

Quality is important here; find products that use Creapure, which is the highest-quality creatine monohydrate and tends to cause fewer side effects, like bloating.

Recommended dose: 8–10 g daily

Magnesium supports healthy bones during menopause by aiding in calcium absorption, regulating bone cell activity, and helping to maintain bone density, which is crucial as estrogen levels drop during this time, putting women at increased risk of osteoporosis and bone loss. Essentially, magnesium plays a vital role in the process of bone formation and mineralization, making bones stronger and less prone to fracture. Fun fact: Bone stores about 60 percent of our magnesium, so it should not surprise us that this mineral does so much to help.

Additionally, magnesium is known to have a beneficial role in inflammation and oxidative stress, both risk factors in the decline in bone density. (This is also great for sleep, so I'm including it in the sleep section, as well.)

There are many types of magnesium. For bone health, I suggest magnesium glycinate or bisglycinate; if a patient is constipated, these two forms can also help facilitate bowel movements. I also like it in topical, transdermal form. In fact, I have seen women do best with oral *and* transdermal formulations.

The current Recommended Daily Allowances (RDAs) for magnesium are way too low. They depend on age and are as follows:

- Females (14 to 50 years): 320 to 360 mg daily
- Females (51+ years): at least 320 mg daily

Recommended dose: I generally recommend at least 550 mg daily to support overall health, including cognition.

Vitamin D plays a crucial role in maintaining bone health by facilitating calcium absorption, and studies show that adequate vitamin D levels increase bone mineral density and reduce fracture risk, particularly in individuals with vitamin D deficiency. However, other findings suggest that the benefits of vitamin D supplementation for bone health are highly bio-individual, highlighting the importance of consulting a healthcare professional to determine optimal intake based on individual needs.

The importance of maintaining healthy vitamin D levels and bone mineralization throughout our lifetime cannot be overemphasized. If we remain low in vitamin D, it can impact bone mineral density, muscle strength, fall risk, immune cell changes, and inflammatory responses. Vitamin D deficiency leads to decreased calcium absorption and, ultimately, the release of calcium from the bones in order to maintain circulating calcium concentrations. Monitoring vitamin D is essential.

Recommended dose: 1,000–5,000 IU, dependent on testing; some women require higher doses that need to be prescribed. Use with K_2 for absorption (a form of vitamin K, which is another fat-soluble vitamin).

Sleep

Nearly all women across the spectrum need help with sleep issues in middlepause. Outside of the HRT recommendations, here are a few supplements that can help with getting enough high-quality sleep.

Adaptogens are natural plant-derived compounds that may help you sleep by reducing stress, balancing hormones, and stimulating neurotransmitters. There are many options, including ashwagandha, magnolia bark, holy basil, and rhodiola, but ashwagandha in particular can reduce the time it takes to fall asleep, prolong the deep sleep phase, and reduce nocturnal disturbances. This is probably my favorite because it's "tonifying," meaning it helps balance overall cortisol.

Recommended dose: Depends on the type and brand of supplement

***Bifidobacterium longum* 1714/Zenflore** is a probiotic and has been shown to offer significant improvements in subjective sleep quality and reduced daytime dysfunction due to sleepiness after four weeks, compared with a placebo group. Recall our discussions earlier in this book regarding our gut–brain axis. Shifts in our microbiome have been correlated with sleep issues, and in another study, this probiotic positively impacted cognition and the stress response in healthy patients.

Recommended dose: Depends on the product. I like the brand Microbiome Labs Zenbiome Sleep, which is 50 mg.

Creatine monohydrate (CM) has been a favorite with athletes as well as the lay public to help them enhance physical performance and muscle strength for a while now, but emerging research suggests that creatine can also help with sleep, specifically sleep architecture and circadian rhythms. New data also suggests that creatine reduces sleep need and can boost cognition and energy while sleep deprived. Translation? Those nights that you toss and turn, or when you have a day full of meetings after a red-eye, this will be your friend. Additional research suggests that CM may help increase total sleep duration, which many middle-aged women struggle with. CM also has neuroprotective effects. The mechanism by which creatine enhances sleep is still ongoing and not fully understood. CM is also very helpful for jet lag; we require higher doses to cross the blood-brain barrier both for sleep support and for jet lag needs.

Recommended dose: Typically 5 g daily, but if you need an extra push for sleep or jet lag, to cross the blood-brain barrier, take 10 g.

Glycine induces sleep primarily by lowering core body temperature, a natural process that occurs before sleep onset, and potentially by influencing the brain's circadian rhythm through its interaction with specific receptors, effectively signaling the body to transition into a sleep state. Glycine also acts as a neurotransmitter in the brain, so it can help us relax and may influence the sleep-wake cycle.

According to sleep expert Dr. Michael Breus, glycine can:

- Help you fall asleep more quickly
- Increase your sleep efficiency
- Reduce symptoms of insomnia
- Improve sleep quality and promote deeper, more restful sleep

Note: Do not take if you take benzodiazepines (Valium, Ativan, Xanax, etc.).

Recommended dose: 3–5 g before bed

Magnesium is not just an excellent supplement for bones, it is also great for sleep. Magnesium glycinate or bisglycinate has been shown to have calming properties that help relax muscles and nerves, promoting better sleep quality. This is particularly beneficial for perimenopausal and menopausal women, who often experience sleep disturbances due to hormonal changes, including declining estrogen and progesterone and shifts in key neurotransmitters like serotonin.

Magnesium L-threonate, a newer form of magnesium, has shown promise for its ability to cross the blood-brain barrier, contributing to better bioavailability. Additionally, in one study, this version of magnesium improved sleep, especially during deep sleep and the REM stage. Participants also noted that their mood, energy, and productivity improved.

Recommended dose: Dosing depends on the type of magnesium. I like transdermal magnesium because it can cover a larger area of absorption. Sprays are good, but a bath soak is nice, too: Use 2 cups of magnesium, 2 cups of baking soda, and 1 to 2 tsp borax in a tub of hot water. Soak for 20 minutes.

Myo-inositol is a component of our cell membranes that helps cells communicate in response to hormones. It's abundant in the brain and nerve tissue, is tied to key neurotransmitters, like dopamine and serotonin, and is responsible for communication and regulation of key hormones like thyroid hormone and FSH. It also helps regulate insulin and glucose. We can obtain some inositol from our diets—it can be found in beans, nuts, fruits, and grains—but if you are finding that you need extra help with your sleep, look into supplements.

This supplement can help sleep in the following ways:

- Myo-inositol helps you fall asleep faster and can help you stay asleep if you wake during the night.
- Research has supported that myo-inositol can help improve sleep quality by positively impacting serotonin and acetylcholine.
- Myo-inositol's ability to increase serotonin receptor sensitivity may be the reason it is capable of inducing sleep as well as improving certain psychiatric conditions.

Recommended dose: 1 g daily

Immunity and Stress Support

Curcumin, a plant-based compound found in turmeric that is also a polyphenol, has been shown to help support the immune system and buffer the effects of inflammation. It can be taken as a supplement or, for example, mixed into golden milk.

Recommended dose: 500–1,500 g daily

L-theanine, an amino acid predominantly found in green and black tea, has garnered attention for its potential to alleviate stress and anxiety. While specific research on L-theanine's effects during menopause is limited, its general benefits in stress reduction may offer relief for menopausal women experiencing increased stress and anxiety. A systematic review of human clinical trials suggests that L-theanine supplementation can assist in reducing acute stress and anxiety in individuals facing stressful situations. Studies also indicate that L-theanine supplementation may improve cognitive functions, such as verbal fluency and executive function, potentially counteracting cognitive decline associated with stress.

Recommended dose: 200–400 g daily

Magnesium regulates stress and immunity and becomes depleted with both acute and chronic stress. This comes in different forms, and I like both oral and transdermal applications to help buffer the effects of stress.

Recommended dose: Depends on type and product

Omega-3 fatty acids have long been a staple supplement for immunity, for good reason. They lower chronic inflammation, support brain and heart health, and enhance immune cell function.

Recommended dose: 1–2 g daily

Phosphorylated serine (PS) is part of our cell membranes; it helps our cell-to-cell communication in the body. It also regulates cell receptors, enzymes, and signaling molecules that regulate the function of our hormones. It is most concentrated in the cells of organs with high demands, like our brain, heart, muscles, liver, and more. PS is very important for modulating the stress response and adrenal health by promoting balanced cortisol levels.

Recommended dose: 1 g, as needed

Vitamin C is a water-soluble vitamin and antioxidant. It helps to reduce oxidative stress in menopause and enhances immune function. It also helps reduce inflammation, supports adrenals, and helps to buffer stress.

Recommended dose: 500–1,000 g daily

Vitamin D_3 with K_2 supports a healthy immune system and helps to reduce inflammation.

Low vitamin D levels have been implicated in not only autoimmunity but also blood sugar dysregulation and poor immune function.

Recommended dose: 1,000 IU minimum daily

Hormone Precursors (a.k.a. Supplemental Options)

In addition to the therapies we discussed in chapter 9, there are supplements out there that can support our levels if we need extra help. In addition to the following, check out adaptogens, discussed in the sleep section in this chapter. "Test, don't guess" is my motto. In other words, before taking these, don't just assume you need them—first test to confirm that your body is indeed in need of some help.

DHEA is an extremely important precursor hormone. It is synthesized from cholesterol through pregnenolone by the adrenal glands and can convert into other hormones, like testosterone and estrogen. Just like so many other things do, it declines with aging. But if I notice someone with low DHEA, I start thinking about chronic stress and see if we can bring those levels up before taking supplements. If not, then we can slowly add in DHEA supplementation.

Low levels of DHEA are associated with low libido, reduced bone mineral density, and osteoporosis in women. Good levels of DHEA are associated with brain health, immune function, bone metabolism, blood sugar regulation, and a healthy libido.

Recommended dose: 5–10 mg daily

Pregnenolone is referred to as the grandparent hormone and is the precursor to DHEA and progesterone. It is also synthesized via cholesterol. It declines with age, like most hormones, and declines under stress as well. It is intricately involved in memory, mood, and sleep as well as cognition. It can be found in our central nervous system and can inhibit cortisol, meaning it can help reduce stress. If it is low it can be beneficial to add to your supplement regimen.

Recommended dose: 5–20 mg daily

Chapter Summary

1. Think of supplements as just that—something that provides an additional (supplemental) boost to an already healthy nutrition plan.
2. Do your due diligence on anything you are thinking of taking. Do research.
3. Consult a medical professional before taking anything.

References for this chapter can be found on my website: cynthiathurlow.com/themenopausegut-references

Chapter 13

The Menopause Gut Recipes

What we eat is so important to how we feel, especially in middle age. That's why I have prepared some tasty recipes to help you on that path to optimal living past menopause. These recipes are loaded with the all-important macros, especially protein, along with fiber, healthy fats, and fermented and probiotic-rich foods that will shore up our gut health.

Asparagus-Herb Egg Bites

Egg bites are a meal-prep classic, for good reason. They're easy to put together and they work as a quick breakfast or lunch—and you can even grab one as a high-protein snack. Enjoy it cold, or rewarm in a toaster oven or microwave. Use a different vegetable-cheese combo if you like; try broccoli and cheddar or spinach and feta.

Prep: 10 minutes
Cook: 30 minutes
Yield: 12

1 tablespoon olive oil
1 medium shallot, chopped (about ½ cup)
Fine sea salt and freshly ground black pepper
1 bunch asparagus, ends trimmed, finely chopped

2 cloves garlic, minced
10 large eggs
¼ cup milk of choice
1 teaspoon lemon zest
1 4-ounce log soft goat cheese, crumbled
⅓ cup fresh dill, chopped
⅓ cup fresh parsley leaves, chopped

1. Preheat the oven to 350°F. Place 12 silicone muffin cups on a baking sheet.
2. Warm the oil in a medium skillet over medium heat. Add the shallot, sprinkle lightly with salt, and cook, stirring, until tender, 2 to 3 minutes. Add the asparagus, sprinkle lightly with salt, and cook, stirring, until bright green and tender, 3 to 4 minutes (if the pan is too dry, add a splash of water or broth). Add the garlic; sauté until fragrant, about 1 minute. Divide the vegetable mixture evenly among the muffin cups.
3. In a blender, combine the eggs, milk, lemon zest, 3 ounces of the goat cheese, ½ teaspoon salt, and ¼ teaspoon pepper. Blend just until combined (don't overmix, which will incorporate too much air and cause clumping). Pulse in the dill and parsley just to mix.
4. Divide the egg mixture among the muffin cups. Sprinkle the bites with the remaining crumbled goat cheese. Bake until the egg bites are just set, 20 to 25 minutes. Let them cool for 10 minutes before removing them from the cups.

NOTES

- You can change the herbs to whatever you have on hand. Tarragon is nice in these (but reduce to 1 to 2 tablespoons), or try a combo of mint, parsley, and oregano. Dried herbs also work well, but use just one-third of the amount. For a shortcut, you can simply use an herbed goat cheese.
- I really recommend silicone baking cups for this recipe. Not only are they the most nonstick, but they also will give you the best texture because the sides and bottom don't brown as much as they do with a

metal pan. You can get them very inexpensively, and they don't take up much space.

High-Protein Maple-Walnut Chia Pudding

Chia pudding feels like a treat but makes for a deceptively healthy breakfast or snack. Just 2 tablespoons of these tiny seeds pack 5 grams of protein and 10 grams of fiber. Combine that with Greek yogurt and protein powder and you'll be full for hours. If dairy is off the menu, swap in a nondairy yogurt. It will have less protein but will still keep you satisfied. The maple-toasted walnuts add a nice crunch and even more nutrients.

Prep: 15 minutes
Cook: 5 minutes
Chill: 4 hours
Serves: 4

1½ cups plain Greek yogurt
½ cup milk of choice
2 scoops vanilla protein powder
3 tablespoons maple syrup
¼ teaspoon fine sea salt, plus 1 pinch
½ cup (80g) chia seeds
½ cup chopped walnuts

1. In a large bowl, combine the yogurt, milk, protein powder, 2 tablespoons maple syrup, and ¼ teaspoon salt. Whisk until well combined. Fold in the chia seeds.
2. Divide the mixture among 4 cups or small bowls. Cover and chill until set, at least 4 hours or overnight, stirring once or twice to keep the seeds from clumping.
3. Before serving, warm a small skillet over medium-high heat. Add the walnuts and cook, stirring, until they begin to toast and become fragrant, 1 to 2 minutes. Add the remaining 1 tablespoon maple

syrup and pinch of salt and cook, stirring, until the nuts are toasted and caramelized, 1 to 2 minutes longer. Transfer to a bowl to cool.

4. Sprinkle the nuts over the puddings and serve.

NOTE

- If you want more maple flavor, add ½ to 1 teaspoon maple extract to the pudding. Whisk it in with the yogurt and milk.

Savory Oatmeal with Spinach, Mushrooms, and Eggs

Who says oatmeal has to be sweet? If you think of it like any other grain, like rice, you can imagine how delicious it is with a savory edge. Instead of plain water, cook the oats in bone broth, which adds collagen as well as glutamine, an amino acid that helps keep your gut barrier strong. Top the savory oats with sautéed spinach, mushrooms, and fried eggs for a fiber- and protein-rich breakfast.

Prep: 15 minutes
Cook: 20 minutes
Serves: 1

2 tablespoons olive oil
5 button or cremini mushrooms, trimmed, thinly sliced
2 cups baby spinach, rough stems removed, chopped
1 clove garlic, minced
1 cup chicken bone broth or vegetable broth
½ cup rolled oats (do not use steel-cut or instant)
Fine sea salt and freshly ground black pepper
2 large eggs
1 to 2 tablespoons fermented sauerkraut

1. Warm 1 tablespoon of the oil in a medium skillet over medium-high heat. Add the mushrooms, sprinkle with salt, and cook, stirring occasionally, until the mushrooms release their water and begin to lightly caramelize, 5 to 6 minutes. Add the spinach and garlic and

cook, stirring occasionally, until the spinach has wilted and the garlic is fragrant, 2 to 3 minutes (if the skillet is too dry, add a splash of water or broth). Transfer to a bowl and cover; wipe out the skillet.
2. In a saucepan, bring the broth to a boil over medium heat. Stir in the oats and a generous pinch of salt. Cook, stirring, until the oats are thick and creamy, about 5 minutes. Remove from the heat, cover, and let stand.
3. Warm the remaining 1 tablespoon olive oil in the skillet over medium-high heat. Add the eggs, sprinkle with salt and pepper, and fry the eggs to your preferred doneness, flipping over if you like.
4. Taste the oats and season with salt and pepper, if needed. Spoon into a bowl. Top with the spinach mixture and the eggs; spoon the sauerkraut into the bowl. Serve immediately.

NOTES

- You can add seasoning to the oats beyond salt and pepper, if you like. Add a sprinkle of ground turmeric, or some Italian seasoning, or anything else you have in the pantry.
- Top the bowl with some hot sauce, or a sprinkle of shredded Parmesan, if you like.
- You can swap in different vegetables if you prefer. Chard or baby kale can sub in for the spinach, or you can rewarm any vegetables left over from last night's dinner.

Sushi-Inspired Shrimp "Grain" Bowls

When you're in the mood for sushi but don't want all that rice, these easy bowls will satisfy your craving. Tossing the cauliflower rice with a little rice vinegar gives it that sushi rice flavor, then you top it with cucumber, avocado, some optional bright mango, and quick-roasted shrimp. A drizzle of zingy miso mayo and strips of seaweed round out the sushi flavors. Swap cooked salmon or even canned tuna for the shrimp, if you like.

Prep: 25 minutes
Cook: 10 minutes
Serves: 4

Sauce:

2 tablespoons mayonnaise (preferably made with avocado oil or olive oil)
1 tablespoon white miso
1 to 2 teaspoons sriracha
1 teaspoon toasted sesame oil

Bowls:

1½ pounds medium shrimp, peeled and deveined, patted dry
1 tablespoon plus 2 teaspoons avocado or olive oil
Fine sea salt and freshly ground black pepper
1 12-ounce bag frozen cauliflower rice, thawed
2 teaspoons unseasoned rice vinegar (optional)
½ English cucumber, halved lengthwise, thinly sliced (about 1⅓ cups)
1 small avocado, halved, cut into cubes
1 small mango, peeled, pitted, cut into cubes (about 1 cup, optional)
1 sheet roasted, salted seaweed (from a snack pack, such as Gimme), cut into strips with kitchen scissors
1 tablespoon toasted sesame seeds

1. Make the sauce: In a small bowl, combine the mayonnaise, miso, 1 teaspoon of the sriracha, and sesame oil. Whisk until well combined and smooth. Taste and whisk in the remaining sriracha if you want it spicier.
2. Make the bowls: Preheat the oven to 400°F; line a baking sheet with parchment. Place the shrimp in a large bowl. Add 1 tablespoon of the oil, season with salt and pepper, and toss. Spread in a single layer on the baking sheet and roast until just cooked through and pink, 8 to 10 minutes.

3. Meanwhile, warm the remaining 2 teaspoons of the oil in a large nonstick pan over medium heat. Add the cauliflower rice, season with salt and pepper, and cook, stirring, until just warmed through and any excess water has cooked off, 2 to 3 minutes. Remove from the heat, add the rice vinegar if using, and toss.
4. Divide the rice among 4 serving bowls. Top each with one quarter of the shrimp, cucumber, avocado, and mango, if using. Drizzle the sauce over each, sprinkle with the seaweed strips and sesame seeds, and serve.

Spicy Asian-Inspired Tuna Salad

This is not your grandma's tuna salad. With the addition of kimchi, a fermented cabbage dish that's an essential part of Korean cuisine, it's funky and a little spicy—more so if you top it with a spoonful of the trendy condiment chili crunch. A bed of cucumber and avocado underneath, simply dressed with a splash of coconut aminos, adds a balance of refreshing crispness to this rich, satisfying salad. Bonus: The whole thing is ready in 15 minutes, so it's a perfect weekday lunch.

Prep: 15 minutes
Serves: 1

1 5-ounce can skipjack tuna, drained
1 large or 2 medium ribs celery, minced (about ⅓ cup)
3 tablespoons drained kimchi, finely chopped
1 tablespoon mayonnaise (preferably olive or avocado oil–based)
Fine sea salt
1 Persian or ¼ English cucumber, sliced
¼ avocado, sliced
1½ teaspoons coconut aminos
1 to 2 teaspoons chili crisp, optional

1. In a bowl, mash the tuna with a fork. Add the celery, kimchi, mayonnaise, and a pinch of salt. Mix with a fork until well

combined. Taste and season with more salt, if needed. (If the tuna is dry, add some of the liquid from the kimchi, or a bit of sriracha.)

2. On a plate, spread out the cucumber and avocado. Drizzle with the coconut aminos and sprinkle with salt. Spoon the tuna salad over, and top with chili crisp, if using. Serve immediately.

NOTES

- You can use canned salmon instead of tuna, if you like.
- Once you've finished the kimchi, don't toss the brine. Use it in salad dressings and dips—or drink a shot of it after a workout (trust me, it's so refreshing!).

High-Protein Beet Egg Salad

For a high-protein, nutrient-dense, delicious, and quick lunch, it's hard to beat this egg salad, which you can toss together in 10 minutes flat with ingredients you probably have in your kitchen right now. Cottage cheese blended with lemon and dill takes the place of mayo and adds extra protein, while beets and celery give you gut-friendly, inflammation-busting nitric oxide. Plus, this salad is loaded with flavor and so satisfying. Scoop it into endive leaves or have it with some grain-free crackers.

Prep: 10 minutes
Serves: 1 (can be doubled)

½ cup cottage cheese
Zest of ½ lemon
2 teaspoons lemon juice
½ teaspoon jarred horseradish (optional)
1½ tablespoons chopped fresh dill
Fine sea salt and freshly ground black pepper
3 large hard-boiled eggs (see note), chopped
1 medium or 2 small ribs celery, minced (about ¼ cup)
1 medium packaged steamed beet, patted dry, chopped (about ⅓ cup)

1. In a small blender or food processor (like a Nutribullet), combine the cottage cheese, lemon zest and juice, horseradish (if using), and dill. Blend until smooth. If the mixture is too thick, blend in water ½ teaspoon at a time until it reaches a thick mayo consistency. Taste and season with salt and pepper. (Yield: Scant ½ cup)
2. In a medium bowl, combine the eggs and celery. Add the cottage cheese mixture and carefully fold together until well combined. Just before serving, gently fold in the beet, stirring as little as possible to prevent the salad from turning pink all over. Taste and season with salt and pepper.

NOTES

- Use packaged hard-cooked eggs to make this quick and easy. I like Vital Farms; the eggs are pasture-raised and they're not overcooked and rubbery like some other brands.
- If you prefer to cook your own eggs, I recommend steaming them—it makes peeling much easier. Bring a few inches of water to a boil in a saucepan. Place a steamer basket on top and place the eggs inside it in a single layer. Cover and steam until the eggs are to your liking, 9 to 10 minutes for them to be cooked through with the yolks remaining a little creamy. Transfer the eggs to a bowl of ice water to cool and stop the cooking. Peel and continue with the recipe.
- Using precooked steamed beets also makes prep a breeze. Be careful with beets, as they can stain your fingers and your clothes. Add any leftover beets to salads, or you can even toss one into a smoothie (trust me on this). Canned beets also work, but I prefer the flavor and texture of steamed.
- If your celery has leaves attached, chop them and add them to your salad. They intensify the celery flavor, as well as increase the vitamin and mineral intake.

Chicken–White Bean Soup

Chicken soup is the ultimate comfort food, and this one doesn't take all day to cook (though it tastes like it did). Rotisserie chicken makes it quick, and plenty of vegetables and white beans add bulk to make this a nutritious and satisfying meal in a bowl. You can swap spinach or another green for the baby kale, if you like.

Prep: 20 minutes
Cook: 35 minutes
Yield: About 14 cups

1 tablespoon olive oil
1 small onion, diced
2 large carrots, diced
2 large ribs celery, diced
Fine sea salt and freshly ground black pepper
4 cloves garlic, minced
1 teaspoon dried oregano
1 dried bay leaf
2 14-ounce cans white beans, drained, rinsed
Pinch of red pepper flakes, optional
3 cups shredded chicken, from a rotisserie bird
8 cups chicken bone broth
5 ounces baby kale, chopped
1 to 2 tablespoons lemon juice
¼ cup freshly grated Parmesan, optional

1. Warm the oil in a pot over medium heat. Add the onion, carrots, and celery, sprinkle with salt, and cook, stirring occasionally, until the vegetables are tender, 5 to 6 minutes. Add the garlic, oregano, and bay leaf; sauté until fragrant, 1 to 2 minutes.
2. Add the beans, red pepper flakes (if using), and the chicken, then stir in the broth. Raise the heat to high and bring to a boil, then reduce to medium-low, stir, partially cover, and simmer for 15 minutes. Stir in the kale and 1 tablespoon of the lemon juice, partially cover again, and simmer for 5 to 10 minutes more, until the flavors have melded and the kale has softened.
3. Taste and season the soup with salt and pepper. Add more lemon juice, if needed. Remove the bay leaf. Divide the soup into bowls, top

each with Parmesan, if desired, and serve. (If you have leftover soup, let it cool completely, place in a covered container, and refrigerate for up to 4 days, or freeze for up to 3 months.)

Balsamic-Marinated Skirt Steak

Skirt steak is one of my favorite cuts—it has so much flavor, and it's super fast to cook, perfect for weeknight dinners. This marinade uses ingredients you probably already have in the pantry, but it gives the steak a complex, rich flavor that makes it seem like you spent hours on it. Broil it, or cook it on the grill if the weather is cooperating. This marinade is also delicious on chicken thighs and pork tenderloin.

Prep: 10 minutes
Rest: 1½ hours
Cook: 10 minutes
Serves: 4

2 tablespoons balsamic vinegar
2 tablespoons olive or avocado oil
1 tablespoon coconut aminos
1 tablespoon tamari
1 teaspoon Dijon mustard
2 teaspoons garlic powder
½ teaspoon onion powder
Dash of Worcestershire sauce
1¼ pounds skirt steak
Fine sea salt and freshly ground black pepper
Flaky sea salt, optional

1. In a large bowl or glass baking dish, whisk together the vinegar, oil, coconut aminos, tamari, mustard, garlic and onion powders, and Worcestershire sauce. Pat the steak dry thoroughly and add it to the marinade, turning it over a few times to coat it. Cover and refrigerate for at least 1 hour and up to 6 hours.

2. Remove the steak from the fridge 30 minutes before cooking to let it come to room temperature.
3. Preheat the broiler. Remove the steak from the marinade (discard any excess marinade), pat it dry, and season it generously all over with salt and lightly with pepper. Place it on a rimmed baking sheet. Broil the steak, turning it over once, until it's cooked to medium-rare (an instant-read thermometer inserted in the thickest part should read 125°F to 130°F), 3 to 4 minutes on one side, 1 to 2 minutes on the other, depending on thickness. Transfer the steak to a cutting board, tent with foil, and let it rest for at least 5 minutes.
4. Slice the steak against the grain. Sprinkle with flaky sea salt, if desired, and serve.

NOTE

- Leave the broiler on, and while the steak is resting, broil some asparagus to go with it.

Green Tea–Poached Cod with Miso-Butter Mushrooms

Poaching fish is an elegant way to cook it—plus, it's quick and foolproof, and it doesn't leave your kitchen smelling fishy. Here you take budget-friendly cod and poach it in a mixture of antioxidant-rich green tea, ginger, and garlic, for a delicate dish that's full of flavor. On the side are simply sauteed mushrooms tossed with gut-friendly miso butter. Add a green veggie or a salad on the side to round out the plate, if you like.

Prep: 20 minutes
Cook: 40 minutes
Serves: 4

1 tablespoon avocado oil
1 pound button or cremini mushrooms, sliced
Fine sea salt and freshly ground black pepper
2 tablespoons unsalted butter, at room temperature
1 tablespoon miso paste

1 teaspoon coconut aminos
5 green tea bags
3 cloves garlic, thinly sliced
1 3-inch piece fresh ginger, peeled, thinly sliced
3 scallions, white and light green parts only, sliced on a diagonal
2 tablespoons unseasoned rice vinegar
4 4- to 6-ounce cod fillets

1. Warm the oil in a medium skillet over medium-high heat. Add the mushrooms, sprinkle lightly with salt, and cook, stirring occasionally, until the mushrooms have released their water and are turning golden, 10 to 15 minutes. While the mushrooms are cooking, mash together the butter, miso paste, and coconut aminos. When the mushrooms have finished cooking, remove the skillet from the heat, add the miso butter, stir, and allow it to melt over the mushrooms.
2. In a pot or large skillet with high sides, bring 5 cups of water to a boil. Turn off the heat, add the tea bags, garlic, ginger, and scallions; cover and steep for 5 to 10 minutes. Remove the tea bags.
3. Place the skillet over medium-low heat and bring it to a light simmer. Stir in the vinegar. Pat the fish dry, sprinkle with salt and pepper, and carefully place it in the poaching liquid (if the liquid doesn't cover or at least come most of the way to the top of the fish, add water or broth to raise the level). Cover and cook until the fish is just cooked through and flakes with a fork, 6 to 8 minutes. Carefully transfer the fish to a serving platter or individual plates, sprinkle with additional salt, and serve with the mushrooms.

Slow-Roasted Salmon with Jicama-Apple Slaw

If you've never slow-roasted salmon before, meet your new favorite cooking method. It's easy and foolproof, and it results in melt-in-your-mouth salmon that tastes like it came from a restaurant kitchen. The slaw sounds fancy but is so simple to put together, with prebiotic-rich jicama, tangy apple, polyphenol-rich red bell peppers, and a touch of heat from jalapeno. Optional pumpkin seeds add a nice crunch to the slaw along with an extra shot of gut-boosting fiber.

Prep: 30 minutes
Cook: 30 minutes
Serves: 4

Salmon:

1¼ pounds salmon (preferably wild-caught), patted dry
1 tablespoon extra virgin olive oil
Fine sea salt and freshly ground black pepper
½ teaspoon garlic powder
4 thin slices lemon, seeds removed

Slaw:

Zest and juice of 1 large lime
¼ teaspoon honey
¼ cup extra virgin olive oil
1 small jicama (about 14 ounces), peeled, shredded (about 2½ cups)
1 small Granny Smith apple, cored, cut into matchsticks (about 1 cup)
½ red bell pepper, seeded, cut into matchsticks (about ¾ cup)
1 medium jalapeno, seeds removed, cut into matchsticks
2 tablespoons chopped cilantro
2 tablespoons roasted, salted pumpkin seeds (optional)

1. Preheat the oven to 275°F; line a baking sheet with parchment. Place the salmon on the baking sheet. Brush it all over with the olive oil and season generously with salt and pepper. Sprinkle the salmon with the garlic powder and top each piece of salmon with a lemon slice. Roast until the fish is cooked to your liking, 15 to 30 minutes (depending on the thickness of the fish and how well-done you like

it; for medium-rare, an instant-read thermometer inserted in the thickest part should read 120 to 125°F).

2. Meanwhile, make the slaw: In a large bowl, whisk together the lime zest and juice, honey, and olive oil until well combined. Season generously with salt and pepper and whisk again. Add the jicama, apple, bell pepper, jalapeno, and cilantro; toss to coat the vegetables with the dressing. Taste and season with more salt and pepper, if needed. (Yield: About 4½ cups)
3. Divide the slaw among 4 plates, top with the pumpkin seeds if using, add a piece of salmon to each plate, and serve.

NOTES

- If jalapeno is too spicy even without the seeds, use a milder pepper, like poblano. Or if you like heat, leave the seeds in. You also could add a few pinches of chili powder.
- This slaw is also delicious on top of tacos, or as part of a Mexican-inspired grain bowl.
- You can leave the skin on the salmon or remove it, depending on your preference. It will not crisp up, since the oven temperature is so low. I like to remove it, then crisp it in a skillet or my air fryer, and eat it as a snack. Definitely don't toss it—if you don't want to eat it, give it to your dog or cat.

Reuben Quesadilla

Turn your fave deli sandwich into a superquick lunch with these fun quesadillas. Smoked turkey stands in for corned beef, and grain-free tortillas made from almond flour bump up the protein and fiber. Cook on medium heat and place the sauerkraut in the middle of the other ingredients to keep it from getting too hot, which kills off the probiotic benefits (the prebiotic ones are there no matter what). These also make a fun finger food for a party.

Prep: 10 minutes
Cook: 7 minutes
Serves: 1 (can be doubled)

Dressing:

1 tablespoon mayonnaise (preferably made with avocado oil or olive oil)
1½ teaspoons ketchup (no sugar added, such as Primal Kitchen)
1 teaspoon pickle relish
Pinch of smoked paprika (optional)
Pinch each of fine sea salt and freshly ground black pepper

Quesadilla:

1 tablespoon avocado oil
2 6-inch almond flour tortillas (such as Siete Foods)
2 slices Swiss cheese (about 1½ ounces)
3 slices smoked turkey (about 3 ounces)
3 to 4 tablespoons drained fermented sauerkraut

1. Make the dressing: In a small bowl, combine the mayonnaise, ketchup, relish, smoked paprika (if using), salt, and pepper. Stir until well combined.
2. Make the quesadilla: Warm the oil in a large skillet over medium heat. Place one of the tortillas in the skillet. Top it with 1 slice of cheese, then 2 slices of the turkey, the sauerkraut, the remaining slice of turkey, then the other slice of cheese. Place the second tortilla on top and press down. Cook until golden on the bottom, 2 to 4 minutes (pick up one edge of the bottom tortilla to check).
3. Carefully flip the quesadilla and cook until golden on the other side and the cheese has melted, 1 to 3 minutes longer. Transfer to a cutting board.
4. Cut the quesadilla into wedges and serve with the dressing on the side for dipping.

NOTES

- You can make a larger batch of the dressing; it will keep, covered in the fridge, for up to 2 weeks. Drizzle on greens, fold into tuna salad, or just make more quesadillas.

- Be sure to buy fermented sauerkraut to get the probiotic benefits. Look in the refrigerated aisle of the supermarket, and be sure it says "fermented" on the label. (The non-fermented sauerkraut in jars in the center of the supermarket still has prebiotic benefits, but the fermented kind has both.)
- Swap sliced corned beef for the turkey for a more traditional Reuben.
- You can shred the cheese from a block instead of using slices, if you prefer; use 1½ ounces.

Protein-Rich Vanilla-Matcha Smoothie

Can't decide between a smoothie and a matcha latte to fuel your morning? Now you don't have to, thanks to this superquick, tasty smoothie. Cottage cheese adds plenty of protein, bananas offer fiber in the form of resistant starch, and a touch of honey balances the slightly grassy flavor of the matcha.

Prep: 10 minutes
Serves: 1

½ cup cottage cheese
½ cup almond milk (or milk of choice)
1 small banana, sliced and frozen
1 scoop vanilla protein powder
1 teaspoon matcha powder
½ to 1 teaspoon honey (optional)

In a blender, combine all ingredients. Blend until smooth. Transfer to a glass and serve immediately. (Yield: 1½ cups)

Chocolate-Covered-Strawberry Smoothie

Made strategically, smoothies can be a fantastic, no-fuss way to sneak in lots of extra nutrients and protein—plus, they feel like a treat. Here, cottage cheese provides protein, along with chocolate protein powder, and the strawberries are loaded with urolithin A, a postbiotic that may enhance muscle health and performance. A spoonful of cacao powder adds more chocolate flavor, plus a shot of polyphenols and fiber.

Prep: 5 minutes
Serves: 1 (about 2¾ cups)

¾ cup milk of choice (I use almond)
½ cup cottage cheese
1 cup frozen strawberries
1 scoop chocolate protein powder (I use Equip)
1 tablespoon unsweetened cacao powder
½ teaspoon vanilla extract

Place all of the ingredients in a blender and blend until smooth. If it's too thick, add a splash of milk. If it's too thin, blend in a little more cottage cheese. Serve immediately.

NOTES

- Substitute vanilla protein powder and omit the cacao for a different flavor. Add a splash of pomegranate juice if you have it on hand.
- You can use nondairy yogurt instead of cottage cheese here, but it will be lower in protein.
- You can swap ½ frozen banana for ½ cup strawberries, or use different berries.
- If you use a nondairy milk, make sure it's unsweetened. If the smoothie needs a touch of sweetness, add a little honey or maple syrup.
- Swap Greek yogurt for the cottage cheese, if you like. Add a small pinch of sea salt before blending.

Berry Date Bark

Dark chocolate is nonnegotiable for me; I have a small amount most days. And it turns out, it's more than an indulgence—it's also rich in polyphenols. I love using it on this date bark, a recent TikTok trend that I've made my own by including nut butter and almonds for healthy fats, protein, and fiber, freeze-dried strawberries for urolithin A (and the

PB&J flavor), and a touch of flaky sea salt, just because. Whip up a batch and keep them in the freezer for your next chocolate "emergency" (IYKYK).

Prep: 20 minutes
Freeze: 1 hour
Yield: About 16 pieces

3 ounces dark chocolate (at least 70 percent cacao), chopped
½ teaspoon coconut oil
¼ cup freeze-dried strawberries
¼ cup runny unsweetened nut butter of choice
1 scoop vanilla protein powder
12 soft pitted dried dates
¼ cup chopped roasted salted almonds
Flaky sea salt

1. Bring 1 inch of water to a simmer in a medium saucepan. In a medium heatproof bowl, combine the chocolate and coconut oil. Place the bowl on top of the pan with the simmering water and cook, stirring occasionally, until melted and smooth.
2. Place the freeze-dried berries in a small blender or food processor (like a Nutribullet) and blend until crushed into a powder. In a small bowl, stir together the nut butter and protein powder. If it's too thick, whisk in hot water a teaspoon at a time until it's a spreadable consistency.
3. Line a baking sheet with parchment. Open each date and lay them out cut sides up on the baking sheet in a rough rectangle, 4 across by 3 down (don't worry if they don't make a perfect rectangle). Place another sheet of parchment over the dates and, using a rolling pin, roll out until they form a thin single layer. Remove the top sheet of parchment. Spread the nut butter mixture evenly over the dates. Sprinkle with the chopped almonds; press lightly to adhere. Pour the chocolate mixture on top, spreading it evenly. Sprinkle with the

strawberry powder and the flaky sea salt. Transfer the baking sheet to the freezer to firm up, at least 1 hour.

4. Transfer the date bark to a cutting board and use a sharp chef's knife to cut into 16 pieces. Store any leftovers in an airtight container in the fridge or freezer.

NOTES

- You can use ⅔ cup dark chocolate chips instead of the chopped chocolate, if you like (make sure they're still at least 70 percent cacao). If you do that, you don't need to add coconut oil.
- Use another nut instead of almonds, if you prefer. Walnuts, hazelnuts, peanuts, or mixed nuts all work well.

Acknowledgments

Mia Vitale: My literary agent, thank you for supporting me throughout the proposal and writing process. I so appreciate your advocacy.

Lucia Watson: My editor, thank you for being so incredibly supportive of my initial vision and seeing the value in focusing on the gut microbiome in perimenopause and menopause.

Kathy Huck: Thank you for all your hard work and dedication in bringing this vision to fruition. Thank you for getting the very best book out of me, despite the craziness of my life the past eight months, and for keeping me focused on the big vision and not the minutiae.

Beth Lipton: Our second collaboration. Thank you for the recipes and tips that align with core principles in the book. You are so talented.

Abby Thexton: Thank you for all your research support during this process.

To my team: Tessa Guevara, and the rest, thank you for providing me with the space to write the past eight-plus months during a year of utter absurdity; I appreciate each of you immensely.

Teri Cochrane: Thank you for always holding space for me in your heart. Your love and support are appreciated beyond measure.

Roseann Campana-Hodge: Thank you for being an amazing friend and for being a safe place to vent and explore ideas with the past six-plus years. Love you, my sister!

JJ Virgin: Thank you for being my mentor, friend, and confidante for the past seven-plus years. Your guidance and support has made such a huge impact on me not only personally but professionally as well.

To all my incredible colleagues and peers who have taught me more about women's health and physiology than any formal medical training could ever do! I sit in complete gratitude for the work you do to not only help advance high-level care to women at a vulnerable time in their lives but also advocate for more research.

Physicians: Drs. Sara Gottfried, Felice Gersh, Mary Claire Haver, Vonda Wright, Carrie Jones, Lara Briden, Corinne Menn, Avrum Bluming, Lindsey Berkson, Anna Cabeca, Amy Killen, Tabatha Barber, Deb Matthews; my sister from another mister, Dr. Stephanie Estima, and Mariza Snyder. Marcelle Pick, Jacki Piasta, Rachel Bonner, and Heather Quaile, thank you for being an example to all NPs and APNs.

Esther Blum: Thank you for your friendship and your ability to provide so much levity to this space. Your grace and humor do not go unnoticed, my friend!

Dr. Gabor Maté: Your work and book *The Myth of Normal* changed my perception of my father and his alcoholism. Our podcast together was a gift, especially given the loss of my father in 2024.

Dr. Lisa Mosconi: Your book *The XX Brain* changed everything for me. Thank you for the incredible work, research, and advocacy you do on behalf of all women, especially those of us in menopause.

Dr. Betty Murray: Thank you for sharing so generously.

Dr. Colleen Cutcliffe: Our interview together got the "wheels turning" on keystone bacteria and the impact of akkermansia, in particular.

Gut health experts: Drs. William Li, Robynne Chutkan, Tim Spector, and Steve Gundry, thank you for expanding my knowledge around the gut microbiome, so profoundly.

Researchers: Drs. Carol Tavris and Stacy Sims, thank you for inspiring me and for the incredible efforts you each go to educate women about their health and their bodies.

To all my subscribers, readers, and listeners, thank you for making this book a possibility; I hope it will help change your life.

Frequently Asked Questions

Microbiome

Jacqueline, 70, menopause

Q: Can changes in the gut make menopause symptoms like hot flashes worse?

A: Yes, unfortunately. There are a few reasons for this: First, shifts in the estrobolome can impact how we get rid of estrogen; if this is impaired, we can recirculate estrogen and exacerbate low-estrogen symptoms (like hot flashes, night sweats, vaginal dryness, and brain fog).

Second, poor gut function can also lead to leaky gut and chronic low-grade inflammation, with specific inflammatory messengers (cytokines) affecting how we regulate our internal thermostat in the hypothalamus. Third, a disruption in the gut–brain axis can impact not only our mood neurotransmitters, like GABA and serotonin, but also our nervous system, as well as blood sugar management, so as we lose insulin sensitivity, our dietary choices, sleep quality, and stressors can worsen symptoms, too.

Andrea, 45, early menopause

Q: I've noticed that I've intermittently had some blood in my poop. What can this mean? I'm not experiencing any other issues right now.

A: Common reasons for occasional blood in the stool can be an internal or external hemorrhoid, eating foods like beets that can darken stool, or taking medications like Pepto Bismol that can darken stool temporarily.

Nonetheless, if your symptoms are combined with weight loss or other changes, I would definitely encourage you to report these symptoms sooner rather than later with your PCP. Hopefully, it is benign and not a cause for concern, but it is always best to get it checked out.

Immunity

Kelly, 42, perimenopause

Q: Why do I seem to get sick more frequently in perimenopause? What am I doing wrong?

A: We have shifts in immune function with changes in our sex hormones, so it is not surprising to know that we seem to get sick more easily, especially if we are not taking care of ourselves. Focusing on lifestyle measures, including high-quality sleep, stress management, high-quality nutrition, and exercise, is key, as well as addressing underlying hormonal imbalances with HRT, if it's appropriate for you.

Heather, 62, menopause

Q: Every stool test that I've had done in the past several years shows I have opportunistic infections like *H. pylori*, etc. I get these treated, but they always come back. HELP!

A: Many things can make us more susceptible to opportunistic infections, including low HCl (stomach acid) and changes to the microbiome that accompany the menopausal transition. I'd work diligently with your internist to rule out reasons for the *H. pylori*, which is transmitted through saliva and sex. Make sure your partner is treated at the same time.

Ovaries

Sarah, 38, perimenopause

Q: I'm not yet in menopause, but I haven't had a period in about six months, and I'm not pregnant. I intermittent-fast for eighteen hours a day and exercise daily; I might not be eating enough food, honestly. I also just went through a divorce eight months ago, and I feel very stressed about it. I'm scared.

A: OK, don't be scared. In rare instances, women can go into menopause early, but not having periods can also be attributable to something called functional hypothalamic amenorrhea (FHA), which is when your brain isn't telling your ovaries to release an egg. Too much stress, too much exercise, and undereating all can contribute to getting FHA.

I suggest going to your gynecologist for testing and evaluation. Your provider can check labs (FSH, LH, AMH, prolactin and estrogen levels, as well as baseline thyroid levels, as a starting point). He or she can also counsel you on addressing your exercise, stress, and nutrition needs at this stage of life.

Heather, 42, perimenopause

Q: How can I address my heavy menstrual cycles without taking the pill? This is all my GYN offered me at my last office visit.

A: There are definitely more options than oral contraceptives, including oral progesterone for part of your cycle, a copper or a hormonal progestin IUD, and surgical options (ablation or hysterectomy). I would definitely discuss the pros and cons of each option with your gynecologist or internist, as well as your preferred approach to managing your heavy cycles.

Bones

Olivia, 42, perimenopause

Q: I had kids later in life and am still breastfeeding. How can I best protect my bones?

A: Great question! Research suggests that women can deplete their bone density by up to 4 to 6 percent while breastfeeding, especially if they are exclusively breastfeeding. But this is not a cause for concern, as most women will get back to their baseline levels of bone density within eighteen to twenty-four months.

Lactation or breastfeeding is an interruption in normal calcium metabolism. While breastfeeding, women require an additional four hundred to six hundred milligrams of calcium a day, and this comes from our bones. Adequate intake of calcium-rich foods, such as green leafy vegetables, fatty fish, and eggs, along with strength training, will be an important aspect of supporting our bones and also honoring our needs for our infants and toddlers. Additionally, supplementation with vitamin D may also be important. If you are concerned, you could always ask your gynecologist or internist to order a DXA scan to evaluate bone mass.

Sandra, 70, menopause

Q: My sisters are taking HRT, but I have avoided it—until I realized that I have osteopenia in my hips and spine. How important is HRT for preserving bone health?

A: Research supports the use of estrogen/HRT for the primary prevention of osteoporosis. If you are later into menopause, I would strongly suggest connecting with a menopause-savvy provider to determine appropriateness based on your own risk factors. Many women require cardiac evaluations, especially if they are more than ten years into menopause. This may involve both lab work and diagnostic testing (e.g., coronary artery calcification scan, CT angiography).

Nutrition

Teri, 55, menopause

Q: I'm menopausal, and I'm finding that intermittent fasting isn't working as well as it once did. I have whittled down my eating window to four hours and, occasionally, I go OMAD (one meal a day). The scale is stuck. I've started eating less and less food, and I'm worried that I'm worsening my muscle loss and I know how important it is.

A: Yes, this is a common issue for many women practicing intermittent fasting (IF). However, it's one that we can fix! I would start with opening up the feeding window, meaning instead of a four-hour feeding window, open it to nine or ten hours to ensure three portions of protein. Women should aim to consume at least a hundred grams of protein per day. To do so, I typically will suggest a "reverse" diet, adding one hundred more calories of protein per day and tracking to monitor both body composition and macronutrients. This may take several months—continue lifting weights and getting high-quality sleep, as well.

Erica, 39, perimenopause

Q: I'm confused about carbs. Why are they so vilified? How can I determine how much to consume?

A: Yes, unfortunately, carbs get a bad rap, but we need to be more nuanced about carb intake. Obviously, unprocessed carbs can be a great option for many women, but it is always dependent on someone's activity level, insulin sensitivity, and life stage. So if you are still experiencing a cycle, you can allow for a bit more discretionary carbs around your luteal phase (two weeks before your cycle starts), particularly during more intense workouts, as carbohydrates refuel glycogen stores in our muscles. Good-quality carbs include low-glycemic fruits, most veggies, and if tolerated, some gluten-free grains, too. Sometimes an extra quarter to third of a cup can make a big difference for many women. Experiment to see what feels best.

Exercise

Cathy, 57, menopause

Q: I am recently recovering from frozen shoulder. How common is this, and when can I return to a normal level of exercise?

A: Frozen shoulder, also known as adhesive capsulitis, is commonly diagnosed in middle age. We don't know exactly why, but we think it is the loss of estrogen and increase in inflammation. It affects 2 to 5 percent of the general female population. In fact, in some cultures, it's called the "fifty-year-old woman's shoulder." It can take time to heal, and I would defer to your provider's recommendations on when to return to full activity. In the interim, low-impact physical activity and lower-body exercises will likely be fine.

Sleep

Lauren, 67, menopause

Q: I have struggled with sleep—falling and staying asleep—my entire life. I am not currently taking HRT, but am curious about it. I've been in menopause for more than ten years. My internist prescribed Klonopin and Ambien, which only help me fall asleep, but not stay asleep. Do you have any other suggestions?

A: Sleep issues are not uncommon in perimenopause and menopause. With that said, many other issues can contribute, including chronic stress, improper macros, eating meals too close to bedtime, blood sugar dysregulation, and poor gut health. Additionally, medications like benzodiazepines (Klonopin, Xanax, Ativan, etc.) can be habit-forming and should not be discontinued abruptly. I would highly recommend discussing your concerns with your prescribing provider and allowing them to take a deeper dive into your sleep issues and concerns. HRT can be life-changing for sleep quality because progesterone is good for falling asleep and estrogen is good for staying asleep.

Nancy, 70, menopause

Q: I've been noticing that I get reflux symptoms when I eat too close to bedtime. I occasionally need Tums. Is this common?

A: First, eating too close to bedtime (within two to three hours) can be the trigger; it can take a bit of time for your food to make its way out of your stomach and into your small intestines. If eating earlier doesn't help ease the reflux, keep track of your trigger foods—often it is greasy, fatty, fried foods, or any food that lowers the tone of the lower esophageal sphincter (LES), like onions, garlic, chocolate, peppermint, or even caffeine or carbonated beverages that cause reflux. Second, if your symptoms persist, I would see your PCP or internist to ensure that there's not another reason for the flare-ups. Finally, sleeping on your left side, which allows for gravity to help move the contents of the small intestine into the large intestine, and maintaining a healthy weight can reduce the likelihood of recurrence.

Stress

Rachel, 41, perimenopause

Q: I am currently going through a divorce and am *super* stressed out. I'm trying to walk daily, I meditate as much as possible, but the stress is unrelenting. *Help!*

A: First and foremost, please give yourself grace. Divorce is incredibly stressful. In perimenopause, we tend to be a bit less stress-resilient, so you may need some additional support. First, discuss with your PCP oral progesterone therapy during the second half of your cycle (this hormone upregulates GABA, a key neurotransmitter that can help reduce anxiety and stress). Additionally, there are some easy ways to bring cortisol levels down, including getting out and connecting to nature (even for ten to fifteen minutes in the morning), cuddling with your pets and children, and doing breathwork, meditation, and low-impact exercise. In the short term, there is likely also value in discussing your feelings with a licensed therapist, psychologist, or psychiatrist to make additional suggestions and recommendations.

Julie, 52, perimenopause

Q: I have noticed that what I eat can really make my baseline GAD (generalized anxiety) levels worse. How can I continue navigating perimenopause and manage my anxiety levels?

A: I would start a food diary to keep track of what foods worsen your anxiety levels. Eliminating processed sugars and caffeine might be a good place to start. I find that most of my female patients in middle age do best by eliminating processed foods in general. Additionally, please discuss the option of oral progesterone with your PCP, as it can be hugely impactful for anxiety and depression symptoms. They can help determine if further lifestyle support or medication may be beneficial for you.

HRT

Caroline, 62, menopause

Q: I had a hysterectomy when I was 54; I'm now 62 and I was put on E2 18 months ago, and it really improved my hot flashes. Is there any benefit to taking progesterone, too?
A: Absolutely. We have progesterone receptors throughout our bodies, and even with a hysterectomy, I still see clinical benefit from oral progesterone therapies. Many of my patients report better mood and sleep while on progesterone.

Daniella, 47, perimenopause

Q: Does HRT cause weight gain?
A: This is a common question and concern for most, if not all, of my patients. When dosed properly and conservatively, you should not gain weight. Obviously, before adding HRT or any medications, I like to ensure that lifestyle factors have been addressed first, which can impact the results from HRT substantially. These factors include high-quality sleep, proper stress management, anti-inflammatory nutrition, and strength training. Every patient needs to be viewed individually, and dosing and strategies should be tailored accordingly.

Emilia, 53, menopause

Q: What are the signs that you need to increase your HRT?
A: Typically, based on symptoms, if someone continues having hot flashes, or vasomotor symptoms, increasing her estrogen patch may

improve these symptoms. Or if someone is taking progesterone and is experiencing bleeding or trouble sleeping, we may increase oral progesterone therapy. The solutions are complicated, and so are many factors that must be taken into account, including symptoms and lab testing, where applicable.

Supplements

Kendall, 46, perimenopause

Q: How do I determine which supplements to take on a daily basis? I feel like the options get, frankly, overwhelming, and I want to keep things simple.

A: Most of my patients and clients benefit from oral magnesium, vitamin D, creatine monohydrate, something for the microbiome, like urolithin A, and sleep and stress support, like myo-inositol or adaptogenic herbs. Many of these decisions are guided by budget and bandwidth. Slowly add in options and monitor how you feel.

Erica, 50, menopause

Q: Where can I find high-quality supplement options?

A: A good starting point is pharmaceutical-grade companies that have high, rigorous testing standards. Brands that I frequently recommend (but by no means should this be considered an exhaustive list) include Designs for Health, Biotics, Xymogen, Ortho Molecular, and my own brand, the Midlife Pause. I personally ensure that we test for gluten and dairy, which, again, can be problematic for many women in middle age and beyond.

Testing

Rachel, 54, menopause

Q: If you could only choose one integrative test for a woman that yields the most helpful information, what would it be?

A: Hands down, stool testing, especially for individuals in perimenopause or menopause, can be incredibly insightful in terms of inflammatory markers, opportunistic infections, digestive enzyme levels, and fat digestion efficiency, among other factors. Starting with this allows me to determine the next course of action (testing, labs, supplements, lifestyle, medications, etc.).

Andrea, 48, perimenopause

Q: What is the most cost-effective way to rule out food sensitivities without going through testing?
A: I would try an elimination diet, such as Whole30, or just eliminate gluten and dairy for six weeks. I find that most, if not all, of my patients are sensitive to gluten and dairy. We monitor symptoms and then proceed with reintroduction, if they desire.

Resources

Recommended Supplements

Here's a brief list of favorite supplement brands and resources that I recommend to most of my patients and clients.

Gut

Digestive bitters: Urban Moonshine brand (many options)
Digestive enzymes: BIOptimizers Masszymes
Fiber: There are many options, but these are just a few that my clients and I use:

- Acacia fiber: NOW Foods
- Inulin: NOW Foods inulin powder
- Resistant starch: Designs for Health PaleoFiber (potato flour and green banana flour)
- Partially hydrolyzed guar gum: Tomorrow's Nutrition Sunfiber
- Prebiotic fiber blends: Midlife Pause PreBioPro Advanced (acacia gum, agave inulin, flaxseed, guar gum)

Probiotics

- Klaire Labs Ther-biotic Leaky Gut (soil-based)
- MegaSporeBiotic (spore-based)
- Ortho Molecular *Saccharomyces boulardii* (beneficial yeast)
- Pendulum akkermansia

Immunoglobulin: Ortho Molecular SBI Protect (capsules or powder)

L-glutamine: Thorne or Pure Encapsulations
Nitric oxide: N1o1 lozenges or N.O. Beetz
Polyphenols: Pendulum Polyphenol Booster
Tudca: BodyBio
Urolithin A: Timeline Nutrition Mitopure

Bones

Collagen peptides: Midlife Pause CollagenPro Midlife
Creatine monohydrate: Midlife Pause MLP Creatine+
Magnesium glycinate or bisglycinate: Designs for Health, Thorne, and Qualira brands are great; as a spray, Ancient Minerals or Beam Minerals
Vitamin D: Midlife Pause D3-K2Pro Complete

Sleep

Adaptogens: Can be taken separately or in a blend; for blends, I like Gaia Pro, Designs for Health, and Ortho Molecular.
***Bifidobacterium longum* 1714/Zenflore:** Zenbiome Dual, Cope, or Sleep by Microbiome Labs
Creatine monohydrate: Midlife Pause MLP Creatine+
Glycine: Designs for Health
Magnesium L-threonate: Xymogen; as a spray: Ancient Minerals or Beam Minerals
Myo-inositol: Midlife Pause Inositol+

Stress

Curcumin: Designs for Health
L-theanine: Integrative Therapeutics, Klaire Labs, Thorne
Magnesium: Xymogen, Ancient Minerals, Designs for Health, Qualia
Omega-3 fatty acids: Xymogen
Phosphorylated serine (PS): BodyBio
Vitamin C: Designs for Health Stellar C
Vitamin D/K_2: Midlife Pause D3-K2Pro

Hormone Precursors

DHEA: Ortho Molecular, Designs for Health
Julva: If you are not able to currently use vaginal hormones, this is a nice option formulated by an OB-GYN and has clean ingredients.
Pregnenolone: Ortho Molecular

Further Reading

Hormones

The Autoimmune Cure: Healing the Trauma and Other Triggers That Have Turned Your Body Against You by Dr. Sara Szal Gottfried, Harvest, 2024.

Estrogen Matters: Why Taking Hormones in Menopause Can Improve and Lengthen Women's Lives—Without Raising the Risk of Breast Cancer by Drs. Avrum Bluming and Carol Tavris, Little, Brown Spark, 2017.

The Hormone Fix: Burn Fat Naturally, Boost Energy, Sleep Better, and Stop Hot Flashes, the Keto-Green Way by Dr. Anna Cabeca, Ballantine, 2019.

The New Menopause: Navigating Your Path Through Hormonal Change with Purpose, Power, and Facts by Mary Claire Haver MD, Rodale, 2024.

Brain

The Menopause Brain: New Science Empowers Women to Navigate the Pivotal Transition with Knowledge and Confidence by Dr. Lisa Mosconi, Avery, 2024.

The XX Brain: The Groundbreaking Science Empowering Women to Maximize Cognitive Health and Prevent Alzheimer's Disease by Dr. Lisa Mosconi, Avery, 2022.

Gut

The Anti-Viral Gut: Tackling Pathogens from the Inside Out by Dr. Robynne Chutkan, Avery, 2022.

Food for Life: The New Science of Eating Well by Dr. Tim Spector, Vintage, 2024.

Gut Check: Unleash the Power of Your Microbiome to Reverse Disease and Transform Your Mental, Physical, and Emotional Health by Dr. Steven Gundry, Harper Wave, 2024.

Super Gut: A Four-Week Plan to Reprogram Your Microbiome, Restore Health and Lose Weight by Dr. William Davis, Balance, 2022.

Sleep

The Circadian Code: Lose Weight, Supercharge Your Energy, and Transform Your Health from Morning to Midnight by Dr. Satchin Panda, Rodale, 2018.

Sleep Smarter: 21 Essential Strategies to Sleep Your Way to a Better Body, Better Health, and Bigger Success by Shawn Stevenson, Rodale, 2016.

Why We Sleep: Unlocking the Power of Sleep and Dreams by Dr. Matthew Walker, Scribner, 2017.

Bones

Unbreakable: A Woman's Guide to Aging with Power by Dr. Vonda Wright, Rodale, 2025.

Sexual Health/Pelvic Floor

Floored: A Woman's Guide to Pelvic Floor Health at Every Age and Stage—a Comprehensive Guide for Women of All Ages by Dr. Sara Reardon, Park Row, 2025.

You Are Not Broken: Stop "Should-ing" All Over Your Sex Life by Dr. Kelly Casperson, Sheldon Press, 2024.

Index

Note: Italicized page numbers indicate material in photographs or illustrations.